山东省人文社会科学课题（2020-SKZZ-68）

中医药文化双语启蒙故事系列

趣味针灸故事
（中英文对照）

主编　张　晶　范延妮　曲宪双
主审　吴滨江

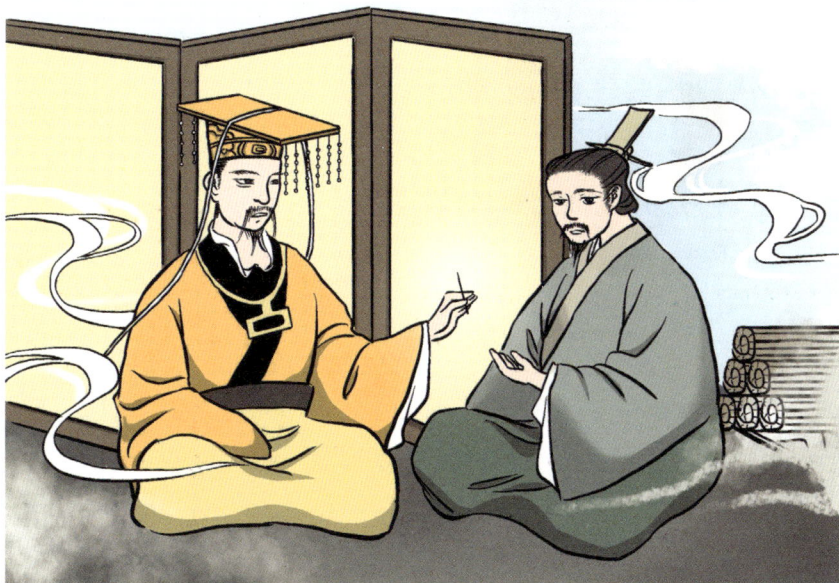

中国健康传媒集团
中国医药科技出版社

内 容 提 要

　　本书介绍了 28 个具有代表性的中医针灸故事，每个故事均用符合现代人语言习惯的文字重新表述，中英文对照，并配以插图。书中以针灸故事为载体，将中华优秀传统文化融入其中，让广大读者在阅读、了解中医针灸典故的同时，也能感受到中华优秀传统文化的博大精深，领悟中华优秀传统文化的魅力，并从中汲取营养。本书生动有趣、通俗易懂，可供海内外中学、小学高年级的青少年，以及广大中医针灸爱好者阅读使用。

图书在版编目（CIP）数据

趣味针灸故事 / 张晶，范延妮，曲宪双主编 . —北京：中国医药科技出版社，2023.9
（中医药文化双语启蒙故事系列）
ISBN 978-7-5214-3926-7

Ⅰ . ①趣⋯　Ⅱ . ①张⋯ ②范⋯ ③曲⋯　Ⅲ . ①针灸疗法−青少年读物　Ⅳ . ① R245-49

中国国家版本馆 CIP 数据核字（2023）第 119209 号

美术编辑　陈君杞
版式设计　也　在

出版　**中国健康传媒集团** | 中国医药科技出版社
地址　北京市海淀区文慧园北路甲 22 号
邮编　100082
电话　发行：010-62227427　邮购：010-62236938
网址　www.cmstp.com
规格　787 × 1092mm $\frac{1}{16}$
印张　8 $\frac{3}{4}$
字数　126 千字
版次　2023 年 9 月第 1 版
印次　2023 年 9 月第 1 次印刷
印刷　三河市万龙印装有限公司
经销　全国各地新华书店
书号　ISBN 978-7-5214-3926-7
定价　**48.00 元**

获取新书信息、投稿、
为图书纠错，请扫码
联系我们。

编委会

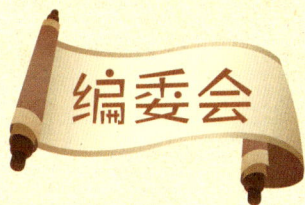

前言

　　中医药学是我国传统医学，为中华民族的繁衍昌盛做出了巨大贡献。近年来，我们国家大力提倡弘扬中华民族优秀传统文化，而中医药正是打开"中华民族文明宝库的钥匙""凝聚着深邃的哲学智慧和中华民族几千年的健康养生理念及其实践经验"。中医药历经数千年的世代沿革发展，内在的文化博大精深，源远流长，为我们留下了数之不尽的动人故事与传说。其中的许多故事与传说，既彰显医理，富有哲理，又不乏生动、有趣，值得我们深入学习并传承发扬。然而，由于中医流传年代久远，很大一部分中医故事与传说分散在不同的书籍资料中，明珠蒙尘，难以被众人知晓。鉴于此，我们在山东省人文社会科学课题资助下，从大量史料记载和针灸古今文献中精心挑选、汇集整理了一部分中医针灸故事，集结成册，以期更好地传承中医药文化遗产，宣传中医药文化，普及中医药知识。

　　本书精选了 28 个具有代表性的中医针灸故事，每个故事均避开生僻难懂的针灸专业术语，用符合现代人阅读习惯的白话文重新表述，以深入浅出、通俗易懂的语言编写成中英文对照的小故事，并配以插图增加可读性与直观性。使读者在阅读中了解中医悬壶济世的传奇故事，充分领悟中华优秀传统文化的魅力。

　　本书在编写过程中，得到山东中医药大学刘更生教授、张永臣

1

教授的精心指导，在此表示感谢！

由于编者水平有限，难免存在一定的疏漏，请同道及读者批评斧正。

编者

2023 年 7 月

目录

针灸故事

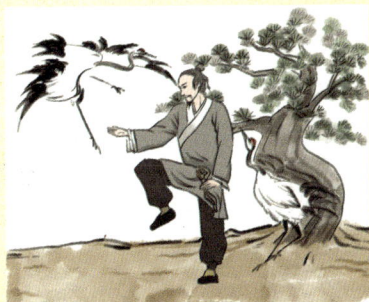

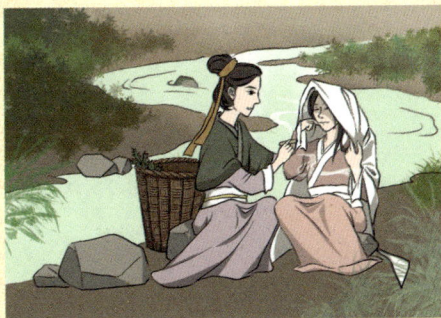

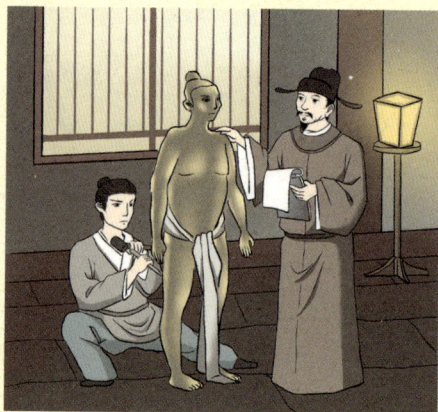

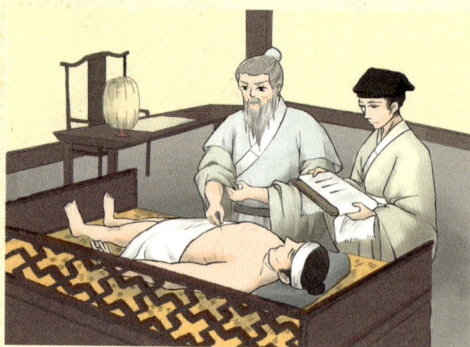

有关针灸的成语

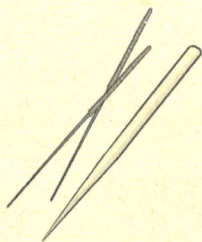

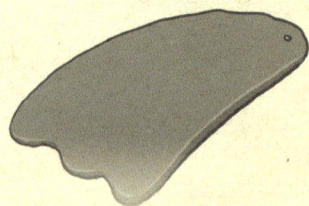

针灸故事

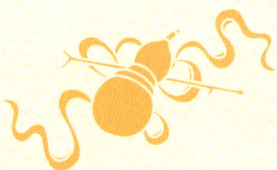

黄帝传授雷公针灸精要

雷公是中国古代传说中的著名医家，他作为黄帝众多懂医术的臣子之一，擅长传授医术，能够通过望诊来诊断疾病，并且对针灸医术十分精通。

有一天，雷公问黄帝道：我在您这里每日用功读书，已经熟读九针理论中的六十多篇文章。年代久远的书册都已经把编绳翻烂了，年代较近的书册也都翻看得有了磨损的迹象。即便我如此勤奋地学习，还是不能理解针灸精要。比如《外揣》篇中讲的"浑束为一"，

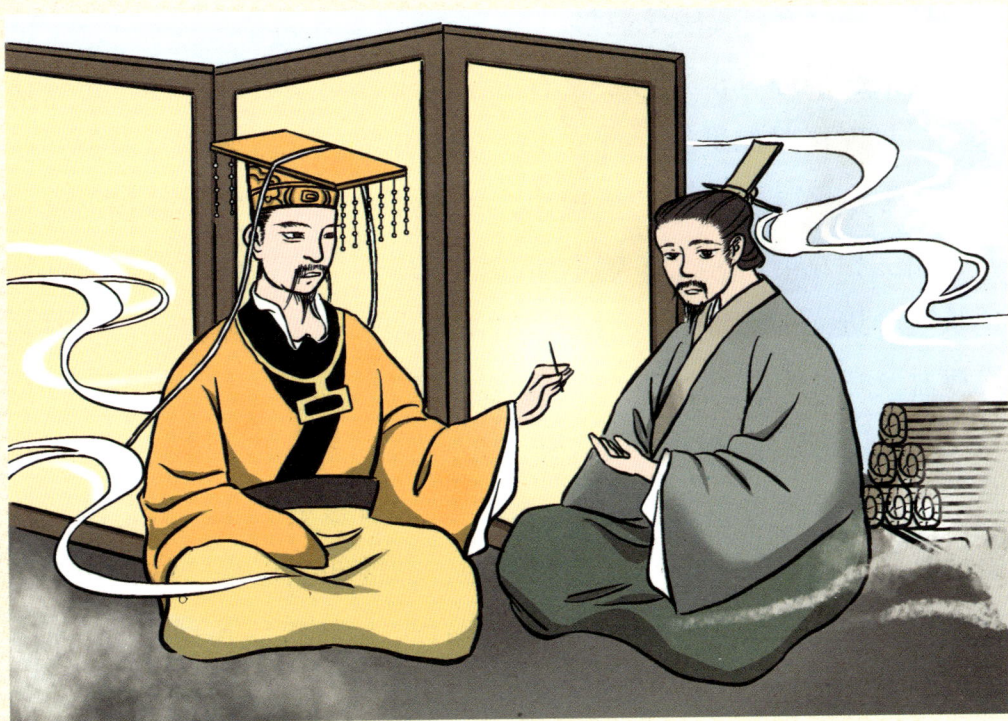

我不能领会这句话的意思。九针之道，大到可以包罗万象，小到可以深入毫微，这样大的方面和小的方面都达到了极致，我不知道如何去概括和描述它。每个人的聪明才智都是不一样的，若是思考得不够深入，学识不够博大精深，又不能像我一样勤奋用心地学习，就更不可能探知九针之道精要之处了。如此这般，我非常担忧九针之道会失传，敢问如何才能概括九针之道的要领呢？

黄帝说：你问得真好啊！只不过这是先师所禁止传授的东西，我私自教授给别人是有罪的，需要割臂歃血的誓言才能够传授给你。如果你想要知道的话，就要诚心诚意地沐浴斋戒。雷公又一次拜礼说：希望您能够传授给我。雷公斋戒了三天之后找到黄帝，表示他已经准备好了。于是黄帝和雷公进入斋戒的房间之后，黄帝告诫说：今日正午接受割臂歃血的盟誓之后可以传授给你九针之道，但是你不可以违背你的誓言，如果有违反，你就会遭受灾祸。雷公郑重其事地拜礼并说道：我接受盟誓。

黄帝左手握着雷公的手，右手拿着书，对雷公说：你一定要认真听，我现在对你讲述九针之道。学习针刺，首先要熟练掌握经脉状况，知道经脉之气的循行规律，了解经脉长短和气血多少；掌握五脏相生相克的规律，了解六腑功能；审查卫气变化，因为邪气都是从卫分进入的。然后，根据病情调整虚实，如果是实证，就要刺络放血。瘀血放出去之后，患者就没有危险了。

雷公说：这些我都已经掌握，但不知道怎么总结要领。黄帝说：归纳方法、掌握理论就像是扎口袋一样。口袋里装满了但是没有扎紧，里面的东西就会漏出来。同样地，掌握知识也是一样，知道了方法却没有及时地整理，等到用到的时候，就不能将道理融会贯通。

The Yellow Emperor Teaches the Essence of Acupuncture and Moxibustion to Lei Gong

Lei Gong is a famous doctor in ancient Chinese legends. As one of the many courtiers of the Yellow Emperor who knew the art of healing, he was good at teaching medicine, hoping to diagnose diseases by inspection method. He was very proficient in acupuncture and moxibustion as well.

One day, Lei Gong asked the Yellow Emperor, "I learned medicine here every day, and I have read more than 60 articles about the nine-needle theory. Books of the ages were worn out in strings and books of recent ages also showed sign of wearing out due to frequent browsing. I have been studying so diligently, but I still cannot understand the essence of acupuncture and moxibustion. For example, I couldn't understand the meaning of the phrase "Synthesizing the Details into One Theory" in the chapter *Diagnosing the Interior by Examining the Exterior* or *Wai Chuai* in Chinese. The theory of the nine needles is so comprehensive that it can encompass everything, and so specific that it can penetrate into the smallest detail, I do not know how to summarize and describe the two extreme aspects. People are different in intelligence, so how can they know the essence of nine-needle theory without deep consideration, profound knowledge and diligent study as me. In that case, the nine-needle theory may be lost gradually in the future. Would you tell me how to summarize the essence of this theory?"

The Yellow Emperor said, "Good question! However, this is something forbidden to be taught to others by my mentor and I would feel guilty for telling you privately. You need to cut your arm and take a blood oath before I can teach it to you. If you still want to learn, you have to bathe and fast sincerely beforehand." Lei Gong made a bow again and said, "I hope to learn it from you." After fasting for three days, Lei Gong came to the Yellow Emperor and said that he was ready. Then the Yellow Emperor took Lei Gong to the fasting room and warned, "You will be taught the nine-needle theory after cutting your arm to take a blood oath. You must not break your oath, otherwise you will suffer a disaster." Lei Gong made a bow solemnly and said, "I accept the oath of allegiance."

The Yellow Emperor, holding Lei Gong's hands in his left hand and a book in his right hand, said to Lei Gong, "Listen carefully! Now I will explain to you the nine-needle theory. To learn acupuncture, the first step is to know the meridians and the rule of their circulation, understand the length and the condition of qi and blood of the meridians, master the mutual generation and restriction relationship of the five zang-organs, understand the function of the six fu-organs, and examine the changes of the defensive qi through which pathogenic factors may enter the body. Then discriminate the syndromes and decide whether it is excess or deficiency syndrome. To treat excess syndrome, bloodletting by needling can be used. The patient will not be in danger if the stagnated blood is expelled."

Lei Gong said, "I have mastered all these methods, but I do not know how to summarize the main points." The Yellow Emperor said, "To summarize the method and theory is like tying a pocket. When a pocket is full but not tied tightly, the things contained will leak out. The same is true with knowledge. If one knows the methods but do not sort them out timely, he will not be able to digest and comprehend the theory thoroughly."

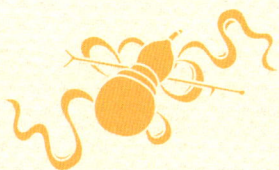

扁鹊针刺太子起死回生

扁鹊，姓秦，名越人，春秋战国时期的名医，齐国渤海卢（今济南市长清区）人。扁鹊是中医学的祖师之一，对中医药发展有着特殊贡献。扁鹊年轻时虚心好学，刻苦钻研医术，认真学习前人和民间经验，并结合自己的医疗实践认真总结。他周游列国，到各地行医，为百姓解除病痛。由于扁鹊医术高超，治好了许多百姓，被当地人认为是神医，所以人们借用了黄帝时期神医"扁鹊"的名号来称呼他。

扁鹊的医学经验在我国医学史上具有重要地位，对我国医学发展有深远的影响。因此，人们把扁鹊尊为"医宗""古代医学的奠基者"。以下为扁鹊针刺虢太子起死回生的故事。

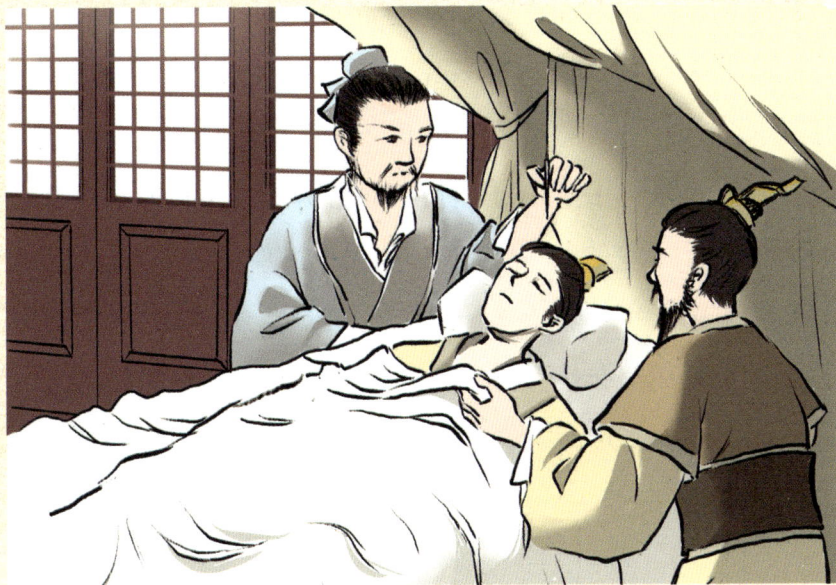

　　有一次扁鹊外出行医路过虢国，听说虢国太子突然昏倒而死，尚不足半日，且还没有收殓。认真了解详情之后，他急忙赶到宫门口告诉中庶子，称自己能够让太子活过来。中庶子认为他是在说笑，人哪有死而复生的。扁鹊长叹说："如果不相信我的话，可以试试进宫诊察太子，您会听到他耳中有鸣响，看到他鼻翼微微张合，沿着他的双腿一直摸到会阴部，会觉得那里还有些温热感。"中庶子闻言大吃一惊，赶快入宫禀报虢国国君。虢君大惊，亲自出来迎接扁鹊。

　　扁鹊说："太子现在所得的病，就是所谓的'尸厥'。人体内有阴阳二气，阳主上主表，阴主下主里，阴阳和合，身体健康。现在太子阴阳失调，内外、上下不通，导致太子面色衰败、血脉混乱，失去知觉，所以身体安静得如同死去一样，其实并没有死。"

　　于是扁鹊命弟子研磨石针，用针刺之术进行急救。他针刺太子百会穴以醒脑开窍，不久太子果然醒了过来。又让弟子在太子的两胁下熨治药物，使药力入体五分，随后太子坐了起来。此后扁鹊又用汤药调理太子体内的阴阳二气，治疗二十多天，太子的病就痊愈了。这件事传出后，人们都说扁鹊有起死回生的绝技。扁鹊说："其实我并不能让死人复活，因为患者本来就是活的，我只不过是让他恢复健康罢了。"

　　通过这个故事，我们可以看出扁鹊医术之高超、医德之高尚，以及中医药临床疗效的神奇和中医药文化的博大精深。中医学是我们老祖宗经过几千年探索总结的经验，浓缩了众多医家的精华，经过了时间的沉淀和验证，有着不可替代的优势，我们有责任传承并发扬中医，为中华优秀传统文化的继承做出力所能及的贡献。

Bianque Brought the Prince Back to Life from Death through Needling

Bianque, who was also called Qin Yueren, was a famous physician during the Spring and Autumn Period and Warring States Period, and a native of Bohai Lu (present-day Changqing District, Jinan) in the State of Qi. He was the founder of Chinese medicine and made a special contribution to the development of Chinese medicine. Bianque was modest and studied medicine diligently when he was young. He toured various states and treated the diseases of the common people based on the medical experience of the previous doctors and his own medical practice. As a result, he was considered by the local people to be a miracle doctor, and was called the name of "Bianque", a famous doctor of the Yellow Emperor Period in ancient myth.

The medical experience of Bianque plays an important role in the medical history in China and has a profound impact on the development of medicine in China. Therefore, he is honored as the "Father of Medicine" and the "Founder of Ancient Medicine". The following is the story of how Bianque brought the Prince of Guo State back to life from death by needling him.

Once upon a time, when Bianque was passing by the Guo State on a medical trip, he heard that the Prince of Guo State had suddenly fainted and died in less than half a day, and not been coffined yet. He rushed to the entrance of the palace and told the prince's attendant that he could bring the prince back to life, but the prince's attendant thought that he was joking. Bianque said, "If you don't believe me, try going in and examining the prince. You will hear a ringing sound from his ears, see his nostrils flare slightly, and feel some warmth near his perineum when touching along his legs." The prince's attendant was shocked by what Bianque said and quickly went to the palace to report to the King of the Guo State, who was surprised too and came out to meet Bianque himself.

Bianque said, "The disease of the prince is called 'dead syncope'. Life is supported by the Yin and Yang from the heaven and earth, with the former governing the lower and the interior parts of the body and the latter governing the upper and the exterior parts of the body. Health is attained by the harmony between Yin and Yang. Now the prince suffers from obstruction between the upper and the lower parts of the body and obstruction between the exterior and interior parts of the body due to disharmony between Yin and Yang, which leads to decaying complexion, disorder of blood vessels and coma. He is not dead actually though it seems that he is as quiet as the dead."

So Bianque ordered his disciples to grind stone needles and applied acupuncture to save the prince by needling the Baihui acupoint to restore consciousness and induce resuscitation. Soon the prince did wake up. Bianque also asked his disciple compress medicine under the prince's ribs to improve the efficacy, and afterwards, the prince sat up. Following this, Bianque regulated the Yin and Yang of the prince with decoction. After twenty days of treatment, the prince was cured. When this story spread, Bianque was thought to have the ability to bring life back. Bianque said, "In fact, I cannot bring the dead back to life. I merely helped him to regain health for he is originally alive."

The story of the Prince of Guo State who was brought back to life by the acupuncture treatment of Bianque, exemplifies the exceptional medical skill and noble ethics of Bianque, as well as the miraculous clinical efficacy and the profoundness of Chinese medicine. Chinese medicine, with thousands of years of medical experience, numerous doctors' exploration and long-time accumulation and verification, has an irreplaceable advantage. It is our responsibility to inherit and develop Chinese medicine wholeheartedly to contribute greatly to the inheritance of the traditional Chinese culture.

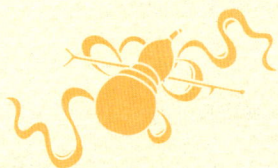

郭玉用针治病精神集中

　　相传在涪水河畔，经常有一位钓鱼的老翁，大家不知道他从哪里来，也不知道他姓甚名谁，只能以涪翁相称。涪翁是个热心肠，遇到生病的人，就主动给人治病，往往能立即见效。他把自己用针石治病的经验和体会记录下来，著成《针经》《脉诊法》。涪翁有一学生，名程高，时常侍奉在侧，许多年后，涪翁将医术传授给程高。程高习得医术后，就辞官归隐，专心行医去了。而东汉和帝时期，有一位很有名的大夫，名郭玉，就是师从程高，习得了医术和阴阳演算之法。因为郭玉医术高超，所以被召入宫，做了太医丞。

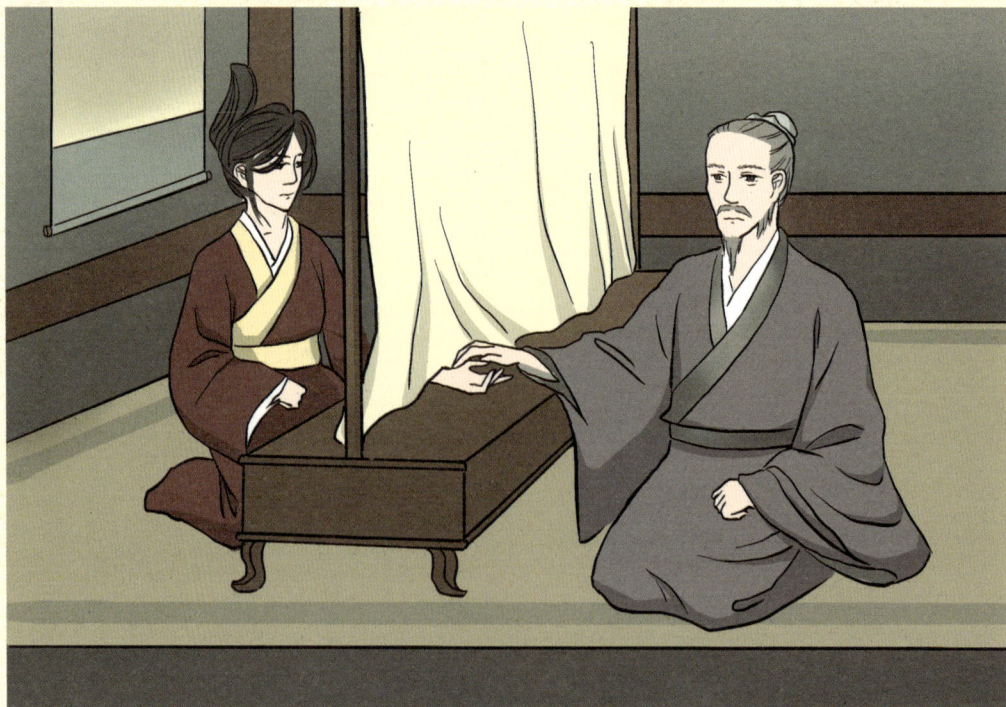

一日，郭玉正在太医院整理和帝的脉案，却突然被和帝召见。原来，和帝觉得郭玉的医术很神奇，于是找来两个人，一个是手臂长得柔美的宠臣，一个是御前的宫女，让他们两个躲在帘帐后面，各自伸出一只手，让郭玉诊脉。和帝说："郭太医，朕这有一患病之人，你看看他得的什么病。"郭玉诊脉后，双眉频蹙，答道："臣诊察脉象，发现左阳右阴，好像有一个男人的脉象和一个女人的脉象，臣怀疑其中有一些缘故。"和帝听后佩服不已，赞叹道："爱卿的医术果然了得！"

在郭玉任职期间，不仅得到皇上的认可，还受到宫中奴仆的敬爱，因为郭玉为人心地善良，即使宫中地位低下的奴仆生病了，他也会尽心尽力地诊治。但是有个奇怪的现象，郭玉给有钱人或者官员治病时，疗效反而不太理想。和帝听说了，觉得很奇怪，于是命令御前的近臣找一个生病的官员，让他穿上破旧的衣服，并模仿奴仆的言行去郭玉那里寻医。郭玉诊察完病情，扎了一针，就把病治好了。官员去找和帝回禀治病经过，和帝听完后，觉得更奇怪了，只能宣召郭玉，问问具体的缘由。

郭玉听了和帝的问话，稍一沉思，答道："大夫治病的关键在于精神要集中，人体的腠理很细微，治病要顺应气血流动，要巧妙地使用手法，用针石治病，有一点点差错就会出现问题。我在为病患治病的时候，需要把注意力集中在心和手两者之间，这其中的巧妙之处只能领会却无法用言语表述清楚。臣给达官显贵治病的时候，因为他们都是身份尊贵的人，所以臣心中颇为紧张，担心出现差错，这样诊治疾病时就不能集中精神了。在这种情况下看病便有四种难处：患者自作主张，不听信我的医嘱，这是一难；患者不注意爱护自己的身体，这是二难；患者身体不强壮，不能使药力很好地发挥疗效，这是三难；患者养尊处优，常常好逸恶劳，这是四难。而针灸治病，需要恰到好处的适度刺激，有时出现误差在所难免，何况我心中有顾虑，时刻小心翼翼，我自己的精神尚且无法集中，又怎么能有最好的治疗效果呢？这大概就是我给尊贵的人治病常常疗效不佳的原因吧。"和帝若有所思，说："爱卿说得很有道理啊！同理，做其他的事情也是需要集中精神啊，这样才能达到最好的效果！朕受益匪浅。"

Guo Yu Devotes All His Attention to Treating Disease with Needles

According to legend, there lived an old man often fished by the Fushui River. People had no idea about where he came from or what his surname was, so they simply called him Fu Weng. Fu Weng was warm-hearted and highly skilled in treating diseases. He recorded his experience of treating diseases with needles and stones in two books: *Acupuncture Classic* and *Diagnostic Method of Pulse-taking*. Fu Weng had a student named Cheng Gao, who ofien accompanied his teacher's side and learned medical skills from him. Many years later, Cheng Gao became a skilled doctor and resigned from his official position to focus on practicing medicine. During the reign of Emperor He of the Eastern Han Dynasty, there was a famous doctor named Guo Yu, who learned medical skills and calculation method of Yin and Yang from Cheng Gao. Guo Yu was summoned to the palace and served as an assistant of imperial physician thanks to his superb medical skills.

One day, Guo Yu was suddenly summoned to the palace by the Emperor He while he was sorting out the pulse records of the Emperor He in the imperial hospital. It turned out that the Emperor He wanted to test his medical skills. The Emperor He arranged one minion with graceful arms and one maid of the court to hide behind the curtain, each with one hand sticking out. Then he said to Guo Yu, "There was a patient here for you to diagnose." Guo Yu took their pulse and frowned, "After taking their pulse, I found the left hand was of a male's yang pulse and the right hand of a female's yin pulse. There must be something wrong with this situation." The Emperor He was convinced and praised, "Your medical skill is really superb as expected!"

During his term of office, Guo Yu was not only recognized by the emperor but also respected by the servants in the palace. That's because Guo Yu was kind-hearted enough to treat diseases for the low-status servants in the palace. But it was very strange that the result was not satisfactory when Guo Yu treated diseases for the rich or officials. When the Emperor He heard this, he felt very strange. So he ordered his courtier to find a sick official, wearing shabby clothes and acting like a servant, and let him go to Guo Yu for help. After examining the official, Guo Yu cured his ailment with just one needle. The official reported this to the emperor, who became even more intrigued. The Emperor He summoned Guo Yu to inquire about the reason.

After hearing the emperor's question, Guo Yu meditated for a moment and replied, "The key point of treating disease lies in the concentration of mind. The structure of human body is very delicate, so we should follow the rule of the circulation of qi and blood, and treat diseases with artful techniques. A small error might lead to accident when treating diseases with acupuncture. I must concentrate on my thought and hands when treating diseases, which can only be perceived but hard to be described with words. When treating diseases for the officials and aristocratic people, I was too anxious to concentrate on the treatment due to their distinguished identity. At this time, there are four kinds of difficulties for the doctor to treat the diseases. Firstly, the patients act on their own without trust in my advice; secondly, the patients do not take good care of their body; thirdly, the patients are weak, affecting the efficacy of the medicinal herbs; and fourthly, the patients indulge in ease and comfort and avoid workout. To treat disease with acupuncture, adequate stimulation is necessary and small errors are hard to avoid. How can I achieve good curative effect if I am unable to concentrate on the treatment due to the anxiety and extreme caution? This may explain why the outcomes of my treatment for distinguished patients were less than optimal. The Emperor He pondered this and said, "You are quite right. We need to concentrate on everything we do to get the best results. I have benefited a lot from your explanation."

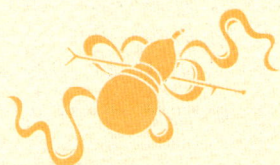

华佗传授五禽戏与针灸医术

　　华佗是东汉末年人，精通医术，拥有一颗悬壶济世的心，并且善于学习养生之道。五禽戏最早可以追溯到远古时代，当时神州大地江河泛滥，湿气弥漫，不少人有了关节活动不方便的情况，古人就想出来各种锻炼方法，这是远古气功导引术的萌芽。再到后来，华佗结合前人的经验，编出了较为完整的五禽戏，世人称之为"华佗五禽戏"。

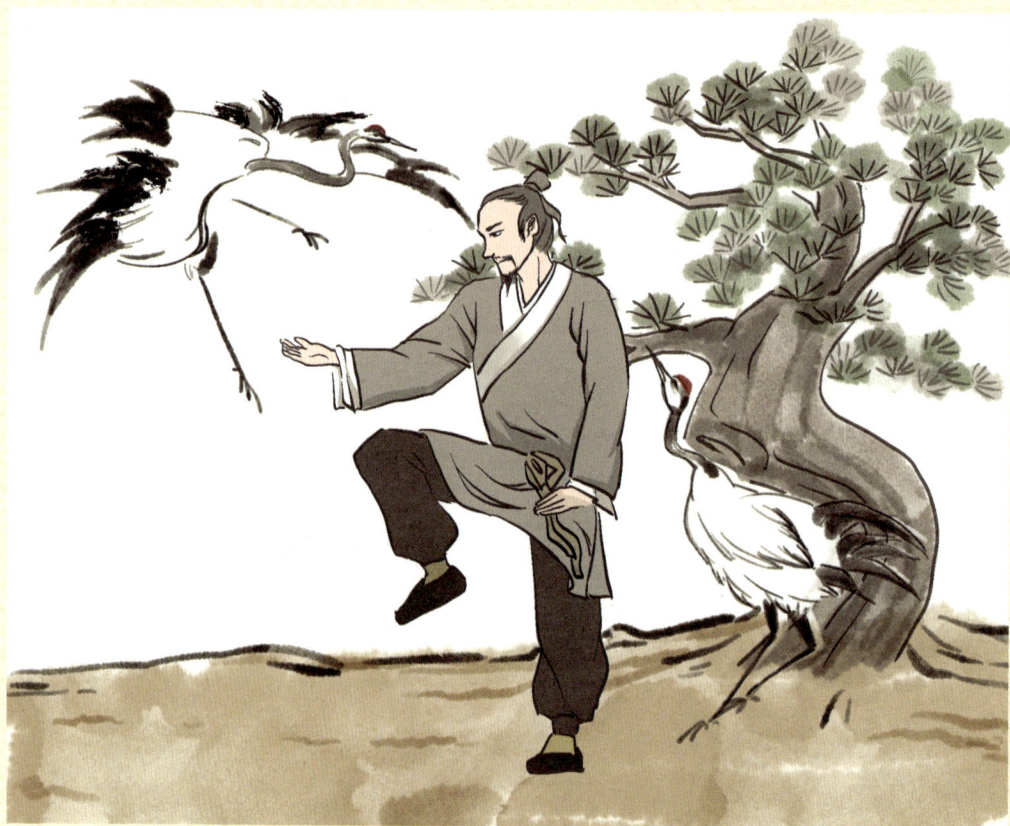

关于华佗五禽戏的记载，最早可以在西晋陈寿的《三国志·华佗传》上找到："吾有一术，名五禽之戏（注：禽在古代为禽和兽的统称），一曰虎，二曰鹿，三曰熊，四曰猿，五曰鸟。亦以除疾，并利蹄足，以当导引。"流传至今，传统的华佗五禽戏主要分为虎戏、鹿戏、熊戏、猿戏和鸟戏。根据梁朝陶弘景在《养性延命录》中有关五禽戏的记载，现简要介绍如下。

虎戏

练习虎戏时，需要双手双脚着地，身体前进三次，后退两次，然后跪在地上，上半身向前趴着，两只手臂向前伸展，同时屁股向后坐，将头抬起，努力拉伸腰部，然后身体向前像老虎一样走路，前进、后退七次。学习虎戏时，要有老虎一样凶猛的气势。通过模仿老虎的一系列动作，从而锻炼人体肌肉的爆发力。

鹿戏

练习鹿戏时，需要双手双脚着地，伸展颈部回头向后看，左边三次，右边三次，然后左脚右伸、右脚左伸两到三次。学习鹿戏时，要像小鹿一样安详和缓。鹿戏主要锻炼人体的灵动迅捷能力。

熊戏

练习熊戏时，需要面朝上躺平，双手抱膝抬头，身体向左、右旋转七次，然后蹲在地面上，双手左右交替撑地七次。学习熊戏时，要学习熊的身体笨重、力气大和性格沉稳的特点。熊戏主要锻炼人体肌肉的力量。

猿戏

练习猿戏时，需要双手像引体向上一样，抓住杆子，身体悬空，再将身体屈伸七次，或者用脚钩住物体倒悬，做引体向上，左右各七次。学习猿戏时，要像小猴子一样身体灵活。猿戏主要锻炼人体的平衡能力及上肢的力量。

鸟戏

练习鸟戏时，需要站直，一只脚着地，另一只脚翘起来，两条胳膊张开做飞鸟状，然后上扬双眉，用力做上述动作各十四次。接着坐下，两腿伸直，用手摸同侧足趾，各七次，再将腿弯曲伸展七次。学习鸟戏时，要身体轻盈，像小鸟一样展翅飞翔。鸟戏主要是舒展肢体，疏通经脉，达到气血的流通。

在日常锻炼中，可以多练习五禽戏，以强身健体，提高抵抗力。五禽戏的修炼应当量力而为，达到微微汗出即可。陶弘景认为五禽戏可以"消谷食，益气力，除百病"，最终延年益寿。

此外，《后汉书》中还记载了华佗针灸的神奇技术，他每次给患者扎针，选择的穴位不超过一两处，艾灸的用量不超过七八壮（注：艾灸治疗时，艾炷燃烧完一次称为一壮）。下针的时候，他会一边行针，一边告诉患者针感会沿什么方向传递，最后应该到什么地方，等到患者说已到，立即起针，病就好了。据说华佗曾经写过一本名为《枕中灸刺经》的书，遗憾的是现在已经失传了。但是华佗的针灸技术并未完全失传，华佗有一个徒弟叫樊阿，这个人十分擅长针灸，并且敢于尝试别人不敢做的事情。《三国志》中提到一个小故事：一般的针灸医生在给患者的胸部和背部扎针时，扎进去的深度很浅，因为再往里面扎可能会因为医生的技术不到位，出现生命危险。但是樊阿敢扎进去很深的深度，并且针到病除。这就说明了华佗的徒弟樊阿针灸技术高超，并且具备勇于探索的精神。

Hua Tuo Taught the Five Mimic-Animal Exercises and Acupuncture

Hua Tuo, who was a native of the late Eastern Han Dynasty and proficient in medical skills, practiced medicine to help the people with benevolence and excelled in researching methods of health preservation. The Five Mimic-Animal Exercises can be traced back to the ancient times when the land of China was flooded with rivers and pervaded with humidity, causing many people to suffer from joint mobility issues. In response, the ancients came up with various exercise methods, laying the foundation for ancient Qigong guidance. Later, Hua Tuo compiled a relatively complete Five Mimic-Animal Exercises based on the experience of previous doctors, which was called "Hua Tuo Five Mimic-Animal Exercises".

The earliest record of Hua Tuo Five Mimic-Animal Exercises can be found in *The History of the Three Kingdoms • Biography of Hua Tuo* written by Chen Shou in the Western Jin Dynasty. It states, "I developed a technique named Five Mimic-Animal Exercises, known as Wu Qin Xi in Chinese (Note: Qin is the collective noun for poultry and beasts in ancient times). The five animals are tiger, deer, bear, ape, and bird, respectively. These exercises can be practiced as guiding exercises to eliminate diseases and benefit the foot." To date, the traditional Hua Tuo Five Mimic-Animal Exercises include tiger exercise, deer exercise, bear exercise, ape exercise and bird exercise. They are introduced below briefly based on the records in the *Recordings of the Healing Art for Health and Health Preservation* written by Tao Hongjing in Liang Dynasty.

Tiger exercise. When practicing tiger exercise, one needs to land on the ground with both hands and feet, move the body forward three times and backward two times, then kneel on the ground, lie on the upper body forward, stretch the arms forward, sit back on the rear at the same time, raise the head, stretch the waist forward and walk like a tiger forward and backward for seven times. When learning tiger exercise, keep the fierce momentum of a tiger. It aims to improve the explosive force of the muscles by imitating a series of movements of a tiger.

Deer exercise. To practice deer exercise, one needs to land on the ground with both hands and feet, extend the neck, look back to the left three times and right three times, and then extend the left foot to the right and the right foot to the left for two to three times. When learning deer exercise, keep peaceful and mild as a deer. Deer exercise mainly aims to improve the flexibility and swiftness of the body.

Bear exercise. To practice bear exercise, one needs to lie flat, raise the head with the hands laced on knees, rotate the body to the left and right for seven times, then squat on the ground and alternately land on the ground with the two hands seven times. When learning bear exercise, get to know the characteristics of the bear, namely bulky body, great strength and calm personality. Bear exercise mainly aims to improve strength of the muscles.

Ape exercise. To practice ape play, one needs to grasp the pole with both hands like pull-ups, suspend the body in the air, flex and extend the body seven times, or hook certain object with the feet and hang upside down. Do pull-ups to the left and the right seven times respectively. When learning ape exercise, be as flexible as a little monkey. Ape exercise mainly aims to promote the balance of the human body and improve the strength of the upper limbs.

Bird exercise. When practicing bird exercise, one needs to stand straight, land on one foot and lift the other foot, spread both arms like a flying bird, raise the eyebrows, repeat the above movements 14 times, then sit down, stretch the legs straight, touch the toes of the ipsilateral side seven times with the hands, and then bend and stretch the legs seven times. When learning bird exercise, remain the lithe state as a bird spreading the wings. Bird exercise mainly aims to promote the circulation of qi and blood by stretching the limbs and unblocking the meridians.

The Five Mimic-Animal Exercise can be practiced often in daily life to build up the body and improve immune system. It should be done within one's capability when there is slight sweating. Tao Hongjing believed that the Five Mimic-Animal Exercise could "help to digest, benefit strength, treat various diseases", and prolong one's life eventually.

In addition, *Book of the Later Han* also records Hua Tuo's great acupuncture technique. For each acupuncture treatment, he would select only one or two acupoints to needle, and apply only seven or eight moxa cones (referred to as "Zhuang" in Chinese) for moxibustion (Note: In moxibustion treatment, the burning out of one moxa cone is called one "Zhuang"). When needling, he would tell the patient the direction in which they would feel the needle sensation and transition as well as where it would end. He would wait until the patient confirmedi the arrival of sensation before withdrawing the needle in a rapid manner with the disease being cured at the same time. It is said that Hua Tuo once wrote a book called *Classic of Moxibustion and Acupuncture*, which unfortunately has now been lost. But Hua Tuo's acupuncture technique was not completely lost. Hua Tuo had an apprentice named Fan A, who was very good at acupuncture techniques and dared to try things that others dared not. In the book *Records of the Three Kingdoms*, there is a small story as this: Ordinary doctors usually keep the depth of needling shallow when giving acupuncture treatment in the chest and back of the patients to avoid life-threatening danger. But Fan A dared to needle these body parts more deeply to cure the disease effectively. This shows that Fan A has superb acupuncture skills and spirit of exploration.

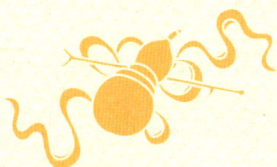

华佗针药并用治疗
将军妻胎死腹中

　　说到华佗，想必大家都不陌生，他是东汉末年著名的医学家，字元化，一名旉，沛国谯县（今安徽亳州）人。人们熟知的刮骨疗毒、五禽戏、麻沸散等典故都与华佗有关。华佗少时曾在外游学，钻研医术而不求仕途，后在各地行医，精通内、外、妇、儿、针灸等各科，尤其擅长外科，被后人称为"外科圣手""外科鼻祖"。他对中医学的发展有着深远影响，后人多用"神医华佗"称呼他，又以"华佗再世""元化重生"称誉有杰出医术的医师。华佗有一个很有名的故事——华佗针药并用治疗将军妻胎死腹中。

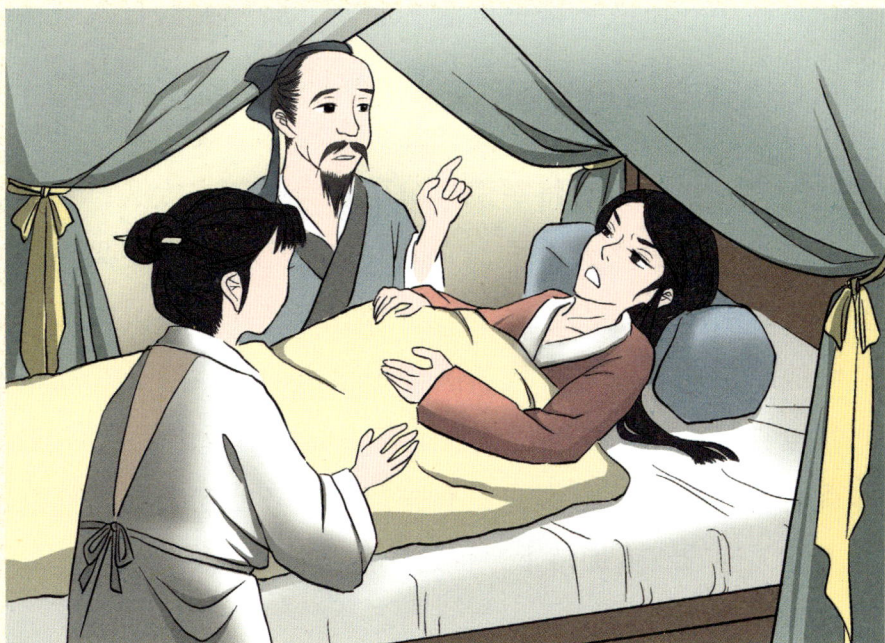

　　相传有一位将军的妻子得了重病，病程较久，将军请来很多大夫治疗都没有什么效果，甚至确定不了所得疾病是什么，这令将军很是着急，后来听闻名医华佗路过此地，便特地请他来治疗。华佗进屋后先是把了一下脉，随即就说这是因为怀孕而导致的疾病，而且有一个胎儿没有产下。将军听闻之后有点疑惑地说："近来确实因为身孕伤了身体，但胎儿已经离开母体。"尽管华佗凭借过人的医术，详审患者的脉搏和腹部，确定存在未妥善娩出的胎儿，然而将军并不相信，且不屑一顾，视华佗为欺世盗名之人，推托了华佗的治疗方案，仅匆匆开了些止痛剂，便将其遣散。服用止痛剂后，将军妻子的病情逐渐好转，但是过了一百多天又复发了。这下将军没有办法了，只好又去恳请华佗。华佗开门见山地说："根据脉象，夫人腹中肯定有一死胎。夫人之前应当怀有双胞胎，第一个胎儿产出之后，夫人出血过多，另一个孩子没有来得及出生，夫人自己没有发觉，其他接生的人也不明白其中的具体情况，没有为其接生，导致第二个孩子死在腹中。血液无法继续濡养胎儿，胎儿死后日久就会干枯附着在母亲脊背的位置，所以夫人常常后脊疼痛。"说罢华佗便开始做针刺治疗，又开了药方。没一会儿，李将军的妻子就肚子痛得像生孩子时一样。华佗又对将军说，孩子在腹中死去太久，不能自己产出来，应当让接生之人帮忙，方能取出来死胎。最终果然产出一个约一尺长的死胎，手足发育完具，但是已经变成黑色的了。

　　这则故事生动展示了古代名医华佗精湛的脉诊技艺和超群的医术，同时也告诫人们，在医疗救治过程中应该给予医生足够的信任，积极地配合医生的治疗方案，只有医患双方齐心协力，才能在医学科技与人性关怀的双重加持下，促进疾病尽快康复。

Hua Tuo Treats the Fetal Death of General's Wife with Acupuncture and Medicine

Hua Tuo, a famous physician in the late Eastern Han Dynasty, with the style name of Yuan Hua or Fu, came from Qiao County, Pei state (now Bozhou, Anhui Province). He is very familiar to us due to medical stories about him, including scraping the poison from bones, the Five Mimic-Animal Exercises, and the powder for anesthesia. When he was young, Hua Tuo left home to study medicine diligently in other places instead of seeking an official career. He practiced medicine in various places and was skilled in internal medicine, surgery, gynaecology, paediatrics and acupuncture. He was especially good at surgery and was called "Holy Hand in Surgery" and "Founder of Surgery" by later generations. Hua Tuo had a profound influence on the development of Chinese medicine, and was often referred as "highly skilled doctor" by later generations. So people also called the doctors with outstanding medical skills as "Hua Tuo reincarnated" or "Yuan Hua reborn". Here is a famous story about Hua Tuo's treatment of the fetal death of a general's wife with acupuncture and medicine.

According to legend, a general's wife was seriously ill for a long time, and the general had sought the help of many doctors to no avail. Furthermore, the type of disease she got was hard to be diagnosed. Knowing that Hua Tuo was passing by, the general asked help from him. Hua Tuo examined the pulse of the wife and determined that her condition was due to a retained dead fetus in her abdomen, a result of a previous pregnancy. The general was puzzled and said, "It is true that my wife's health has suffered due to pregnancy recently, but the fetus has already been born."

Although Hua Tuo, with his superb diagnostic skills of pulse-taking and palpation, identified the existence of the undelivered fetus, the general did not believe him and even regarded him as a deceiver. He refused the treatment suggested by Hua Tuo and sent him away after receiving some pain-relieving formulas. The general's wife felt better at first. But after more than a hundred days, she fell ill again. The general had to invite Hua Tuo back to treat his wife. Hua Tuo said bluntly, "There must be a dead fetus in your wife's body based on her pulse manifestation. She was pregnant with twins and the second fetus was not delivered in time because she bled profusely after the birth of the first fetus. She was not aware of this and the midwives were also unaware, resulting in a failure to delivery of the second baby, which became a dead dried fetus attached to the mother's backbone due to shortage of nourishment from the blood. That is the reason why she often suffers from pain in the back." After saying this, Hua Tuo began to treat her with acupuncture and medicinal drugs. Soon, the general's wife cried painfully just like giving birth to a baby. Hua Tuo told the general to invite the midwife for help because the dead fetus was unable to be delivered by the wife herself. A one-foot-long dead fetus was taken out finally, with its hands and feet fully developed but in black.

This story displays vividly the exquisite pulse-taking skill and superb medical skill of the ancient famous doctor Hua Tuo. It also tells us that we should trust the doctor's diagnosis reverently and cooperate with the doctor's treatment proactively. The disease can only be cured quickly with the combined efforts of the doctor and the patient, supported by medical technology and humanistic care.

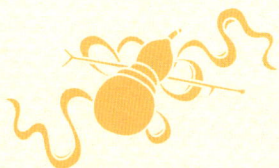

曹操悔杀华佗

曹操被头风病折磨很久了，每次头风发作时都会心烦意乱、头晕目眩。曹操听说华佗医术精湛，闻名遐迩，于是就召见华佗，让他侍奉在自己身边，为自己治病。华佗为他诊病后，用针灸针刺了膈俞穴，曹操的病当即就好了。

后来，曹操料理国事，操劳过度，头风病更加严重了，于是又让华佗为他医治。华佗看过后说："这病短时间内治不好，需要长时间坚持针灸治疗，才能保住性命。"

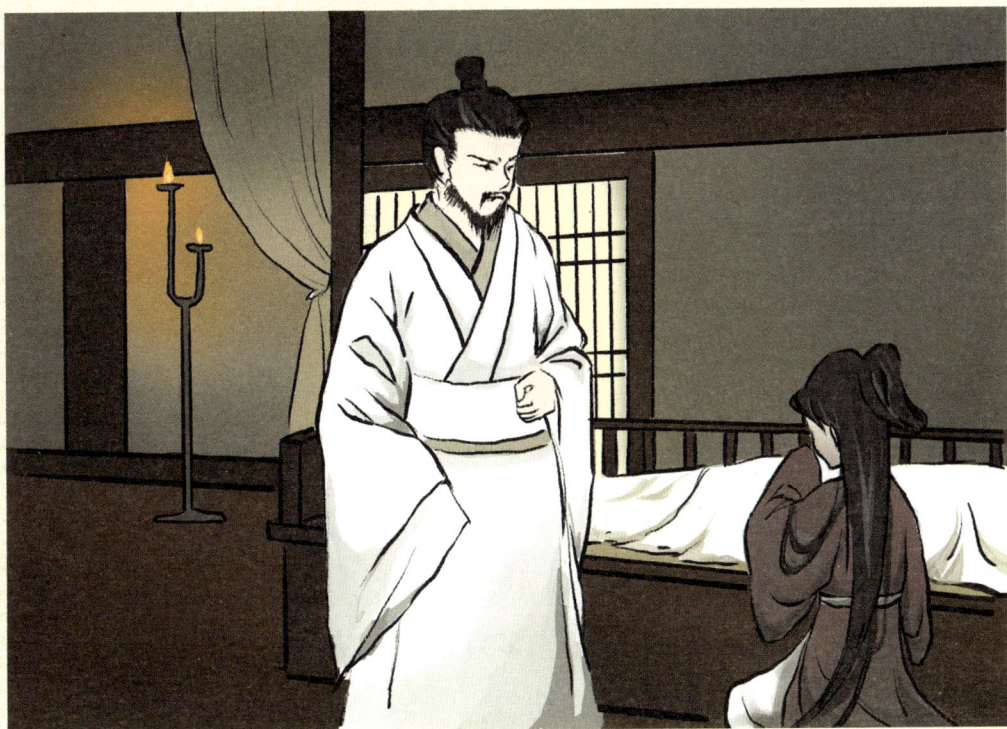

华佗跟在曹操身边一段时间后，非常想念家乡，想要回家探望，于是说："我收到了家里来的书信，要回家一段时间。"曹操念在他治病有功，给他准假，放他回家。到家之后，华佗又用妻子得病为借口，超过假期期限不回来。曹操多次写信催促，还派当地的官员去催他上路，但华佗仍然不肯上路返回。曹操知道后非常愤怒，派人前去查明其妻子是不是真的生病。如果他的妻子确实病了，就赐给他红小豆四十斛（注：斛为古代量器名，也是容量单位，一斛本为十斗，后来改为五斗），宽限他的假期时间；如果他妻子没生病，而华佗是在说谎，就派人把他羁押回来。

曹操的手下去查看后，发现华佗的妻子并没有生病，于是就把华佗押送到了许昌监狱（当时曹操都城所在地为许昌），拷打核实真相后，华佗认罪了。荀彧向曹操劝谏说："华佗的医术实在是高超，与人的性命息息相关，您应该宽恕他。"曹操说："不用忧愁，天下这么多人，难道没有像他一样医术高明的医生吗？华佗这个小人有能力治好我的病，但他不想给我彻底治好，我每次发作只能请他治病，借此显得他自己很重要，若我不杀他，他也不会为我去除这个病根。"最终华佗在狱中被处死。华佗临死前，拿出一本医书想交给狱卒，说："这本书可以救人。"狱卒怕受到牵连，没有收，华佗也不强求，用火把书烧掉了。华佗死后，曹操头风的病根没有治好，再次发作了，而唯一能治好这病的华佗已经死在狱中了。

后来，曹操最喜爱的儿子曹冲得了重病，曹操找遍了医生都没能治好曹冲的病。曹冲死后，曹操很后悔，感慨地说："我后悔杀了华佗，如果他还活着，我儿子就不会白白死了。"

从这个故事能够看出，曹操多疑的性格让他坚信华佗不是诚心为自己治病，没有听从属下的劝告，一怒之下处死了华佗。华佗一死，曹操今后免不了要忍受头风之苦，他年仅十三岁的儿子——神童曹冲就这样断送了性命。那么，华佗为什么不想回去给曹操治疗疾病呢？是真的凭借医学才能抬高自己身价吗？事实上，华佗不想回到曹操身边是因为他不想成为曹操的专职医生，他认为作为医生应当为众多百姓解除疾病的困扰，而不是专门服务于曹操一人。

华佗医术高超，现仍然用"华佗在世"来形容一个医生医术的高超。然而遗憾的是，华佗医术大部分都失传了，只有少部分由他的弟子吴普和樊阿传承下来，两人均成为当时有名的医生。

从曹操身上可以认识到，做人要宽容大度，要善于听取他人的意见。从华佗身上可以看到，行医之人，应当胸怀天下，为民祛疾，方显仁医本色。

Cao Cao Regretted Killing Hua Tuo

Cao Cao had been suffering from intermittent headache for a long time, which made him feel annoyed, perplexed and dizzy every time. Hearing that Hua Tuo was famous for his excellent medical skills, he summoned Hua Tuo to his side to treat his disease. After diagnosing Cao Cao, Hua Tuo cured his disease immediately by needling the Geshu acupoint.

Later, the intermittent headache of Cao Cao became worsened due to his overwork with national affairs. He asked Hua Tuo to treat his disease. Hua Tuo said, "This disease cannot be cured in a short time. It needs acupuncture treatment for a long time in order to save your life."

After spending some time with Cao Cao, Hua Tuo missed his hometown very much and wanted to go home for a visit. He said to Cao Cao, "I received a letter from my family, so I need to go home for some time." Thinking that Hua Tuo had performed meritorious service to him, Cao Cao agreed to grant him leave. After returning home, Hua Tuo was reluctant to come back, so he used the disease of his wife as an excuse, staying at home overdue. Cao Cao wrote many letters and sent local officials to urge Hua Tuo back, but Hua Tuo refused. Cao Cao was very angry and sent someone to find out whether his wife was really ill or not. Cao Cao ordered that if his wife was indeed ill, give him forty Hu of red beans (Note: Hu is an ancient measuring vessel and a unit of capacity as well. One Hu equals ten Dou initially, then five Dou later), and extend his vacation time. However, if his wife was not ill, which meant Hua Tuo was lying, bring him back forcefully in custody.

Later, it was investigated that Hua Tuo's wife was not ill, so Hua Tuo was sent to Xuchang prison (Xuchang was the place where Cao Cao established the capital of his state). In prison, Hua Tuo was tortured in an attempt to force a confession. Xun Yu persuaded Cao Cao, "You should forgive him for his superb medical skills that could save people's lives." Cao Cao said, "Don't worry. Isn't there a doctor in the world as skillful as Hua Tuo? He is a base person for the fact that he was capable of curing my disease completely, yet he chose not to. I was compelled to seek help from him every time I suffered, which made him seem important. He would not cure my disease even if I did not kill him." Hua Tuo was eventually sentenced to death in prison. Before the death penalty, Hua Tuo took out a medical book and wanted to give it to a jailer, saying, "This book can be used to save lives." But the jailer did not take the book with fear of being implicated. Hua Tuo did not force him and burned the book. After Hua Tuo's death, Cao Cao's intermittent headache recurred again but Hua Tuo, the only physician who could treat this disease, had died in prison.

Later, Cao Chong, Cao Cao's favorite son, fell seriously ill and was not cured even Cao Cao had consulted all doctors available. After Cao Chong's death, Cao Cao felt regretful and said, "I regret the decision to have Hua Tuo killed. If he were alive, my son would not have died."

This story shows that Cao Cao's paranoid personality led him to doubt Hua Tuo's sincerity in treating his illness, ultimately causing him to ignore the advice of his subordinates and put Hua Tuo to death in a fit of anger. The consequence is that Cao Cao had to suffer from intermittent headache miserably, and his thirteen-year-old son, a brilliant child, lost his life. Why didn't Hua Tuo want to go back and treat disease for Cao Cao? Is it true that he wanted to raise his price with medical skills? In fact, the reason for Hua Tuo's unwillingness to return to Cao Cao is that he did not want to become Cao Cao's personal doctor. He believed that as a doctor, he should treat diseases for more common people instead of serving Cao Cao alone.

Hua Tuo was famous for his excellent medical skills. Nowadays, we still use "Hua Tuo reincarnated" to describe a highly-skilled doctor. Unfortunately, most of Hua Tuo's medical skills were lost. Only a small part was passed down by his students Wu Pu and Fan A, who both became famous doctors at that time.

We can learn from Cao Cao in this story that one should be tolerant and good at listening to the opinions of others. From Hua Tuo in the story, we can learn that, as a doctor, one should bear the nation in the mind, dispel diseases for the people, and display the original virtue of "benevolence medicine".

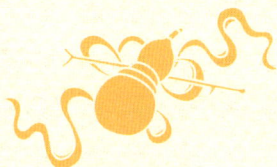

皇甫谧著《针灸甲乙经》

　　皇甫谧，安定朝那（今甘肃灵台县）人，生于公元 215 年，卒于公元 282 年，字士安，幼名静，自号玄晏先生。皇甫谧是我国历史上著名学者，在医学、史学和文学方面均颇有建树。

　　皇甫谧出身东汉时期的名门望族，后来家道中落。在他出生后不久母亲就去世了，因此被过继给了叔父，十五岁时跟着叔父一家搬迁至新安（今河南新安县）生活。皇甫谧的童年和少年均是在战乱中度过。他小时候比较贪玩，和村子里的小孩一起把荆棘条编成盾牌的样子，把棍子当成矛，分成两阵打仗嬉戏。到了二十岁的时

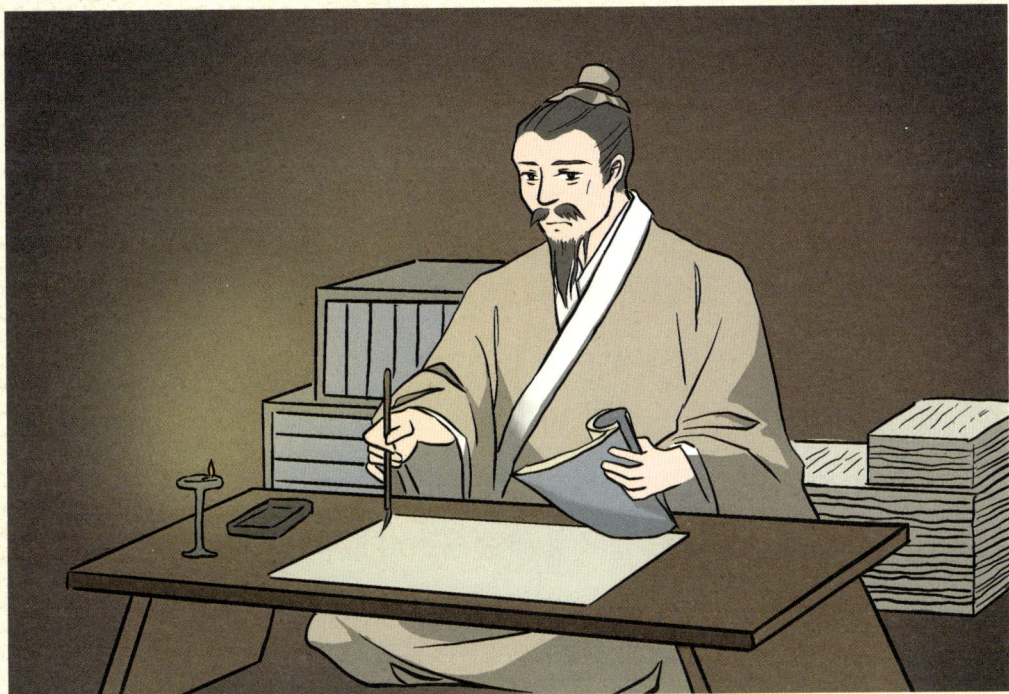

候，皇甫谧仍然整日像孩童一样东游西晃，只知道玩闹，同乡的人以为他是天生痴笨。皇甫谧虽然贪玩，却是一个孝顺的孩子。有一天，他偶然得到了一些美味的水果，就兴冲冲地跑去献给叔母，但叔母见了他不仅不开心，反而掩面流泪。皇甫谧着急地询问原因。叔母说："你今年已经二十岁了，仍然不学无术，就算是再孝顺，也不能让我宽心。古时候有孟母三迁以培养孟子仁义的品格。你如今这样愚钝，难道是我在选择邻居时没有三思而后行吗？还是我对你的教育不够呢？"叔母说到这些话的时候痛哭流涕，让皇甫谧心里万分羞愧。自此之后，他便下定决心跟着乡里的私塾认真读书。

皇甫谧从此幡然醒悟，奋发读书，却在 42 岁左右患上风痹。他在服用中药无效之后，就开始依据《黄帝内经》钻研针灸技术，并尝试在自己身上扎针。他发现《黄帝内经》中还是有不少不够完善的地方，故想重新编撰针灸医书。当时的书籍都是用木简制成的，并且被当作是很珍稀又十分昂贵的东西，普通人得到书籍需要费很大的力气。值得庆幸的是，皇甫谧并没有向困难低头，他多方想办法，凭着百折不挠的精神，找到了许多医书，获取了大量的资料，并取其精华，去其糟粕，推陈出新，革故鼎新，结合自己的治疗经验，编写成了《黄帝三部针灸甲乙经》，也被称为《针灸甲乙经》。《针灸甲乙经》是针灸学领域的集大成之作，奠定了中医针灸学科的理论基础，它作为我国目前保存下来的第一部针灸学专著，影响深远，在针灸学历史上具有不可替代的重要作用。

从这个故事我们了解到皇甫谧在叔母的劝导下，在 20 岁时浪子回头，悬崖勒马，开始研究经义和医书，并取得了重大成就。

Huangfu Mi Authored *A-B Classic of Acupuncture and Moxibustion*

Huangfu Mi (215—282 AD), with the styled name of Shian, juvenile name of Jing and self-name of Mr. Xuan Yan, is a native of Anding county, Chaona prefecture (now Lingtai county, Gansu province). As a famous scholar in Chinese history, Huangfu Mi achieved great success in medicine, historical science and literature.

Huangfu Mi was born from a prestigious family in the Eastern Han Dynasty, but his family's status declined over time. His mother died after he was born. He was adopted by his uncle. At the age of fifteen, he moved to Xin'an (now Xin'an county, Henan province) with his uncle, where he spent his childhood in the midst of war. Huangfu Mi was fond of play when he was a child, often playing games together with the village children in two parties after weaving shield from brambles and taking sticks as spears. When he was twenty years old, Huangfu Mi still wandered around like a child, leading the villagers to believe that he was born with a lack of intelligence. Despite his inclination for play, Huangfu Mi remained a filial child at heart. One day, he happened to get some delicious fruits and took them to his aunt excitedly. But his aunt hid her face and wept sadly instead of being happy. Huangfu Mi asked her the reason anxiously. His aunt said, "You have now reached twenty years old this year, yet you still lack in learning and skills. I cannot be reassured even though you are very filial. In ancient times, there was the story of Mencius' mother moving their residence three times to cultivate the benevolent character of Mencius. Is it because I didn't think twice before choosing a proper neighbors, or I did not guide you appropriately that you are slow-witted like this now?" His aunt cried bitterly when saying these words, which made Huangfu Mi so guilty and ashamed that since then, he was determined to study seriously in the private school of the village.

Huangfu Mi was changed and started to work hard ever since. However, he suffered from wind arthralgia at the age of 42. He began to study acupuncture techniques based on *Huangdis Neijing* and tried to needle himself after finding herbal medicine useless. He found that there were still some inadequate statements in *Huangdi Neijing,* so he wanted to compile a new medical book on acupuncture and moxibustion. At that time, books were made of wooden slips and considered very precious and expensive. It was very hard for ordinary people to get access to them. Fortunately, Huangfu Mi did not give up. He tried every means persistently to search and get many medical books and materials. Then he took the essence and discarded the dregs, brought forth the new through the old, and reformed the set rules to create new ones. Finally, he compiled *Huangdi's Three Sections of A-B Classic of Acupuncture and Moxibustion* based on the previous books and his clinical experience, which is also called *A-B Classic of Acupuncture and Moxibustion.* As the first treatise on acupuncture and moxibustion extant in China, this book serves as a masterpiece in this field, laying the theoretical foundation for acupuncture and moxibustion in TCM and possessing an irreplaceable role in the history of acupuncture and moxibustion.

From this story we learned that Huangfu Mi, with the advice and persuasion of his aunt, returned to the fold and pulled himself back before it is too late at the age of 20 when he began to study classics and medical books. He made significant achievements finally.

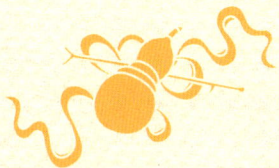

鲍姑擅长灸法治病

在现代日常生活中，艾灸是一种常用的治病和保健强身的手段。灸法治病在我国历史悠久，从古至今，医家们在不断地医疗实践中，探索总结出许多的灸法治病规律。据现有资料记载，鲍姑是我国第一个用艾灸治病的医家。她自幼喜爱钻研医术，精研药理，擅长用灸法治疗多种疾病。如《鲍姑祠记》中所记述："鲍姑用越岗天然之艾，以灸人身赘疣，一灼即消除无有，历年久而所惠多。"这讲的就是鲍姑用灸法治疗赘瘤的故事。

金秋十月，丰收的喜悦洋溢在每个人的脸上，但在越秀山的一个小村庄，一位名叫秀秀的年轻姑娘心情却很苦闷，经常独自流泪。有一天，秀秀正独自躲在河边，一边看着水中自己的倒影，一边难过地喃喃自语："大家为什么都要嘲笑我呢？难道因为我脸上长了这么多黑褐色的赘瘤，就再也不能找到我的意中人了吗？我好难

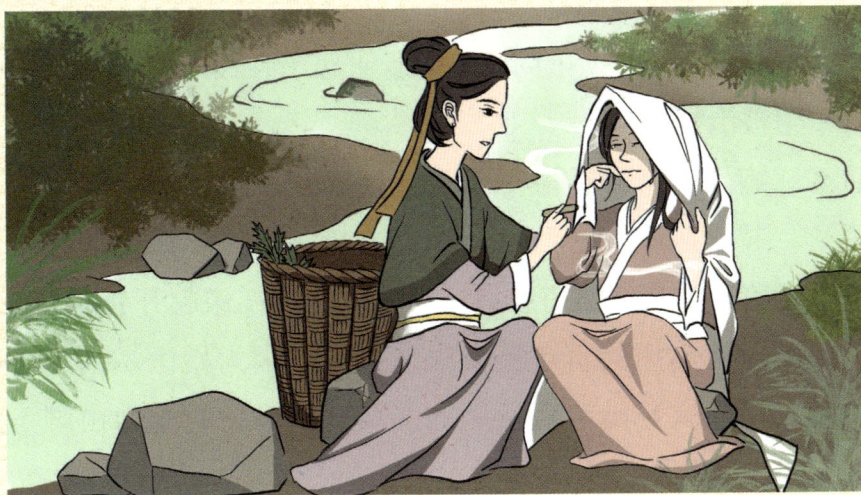

过……如果，我脸上没有了赘瘤，大家就不会嘲笑我了吧。"

恰巧此时，鲍姑刚采完药，经过河边，听到了秀秀的哭诉。鲍姑走到秀秀的身旁，递给她一个手帕，说道："姑娘，不要为别人的嘲笑伤心了，生病了也不是你的错，不要为此而难过了。在我看来，事情还没有那么糟糕，我是一名大夫，平时喜爱钻研医术，我或许有办法能治好你脸上的赘瘤。"

秀秀惊喜地看着鲍姑问："真的吗？真的吗？您真的能治好我脸上的赘瘤？"

鲍姑说："嗯，不过，姑娘你先不要这么激动，我先看看你的病情。"

鲍姑仔细地诊察完秀秀的病情，心中已经有了办法，她一边从随身携带的药囊中拿出一些红脚艾，一边对秀秀说："姑娘，你放心吧，我有方法能解决你的烦恼。"

只见鲍姑把红脚艾搓成艾绒，然后将搓好的艾绒点燃，轻轻地在秀秀的脸上进行熏灼，并叮嘱道："如果有不舒服就和我说。"秀秀小声答应，心中既忐忑又期待。

艾绒燃烧完后，鲍姑又仔细察看了一下秀秀脸上的赘瘤，说："这次的治疗已经结束了，你脸上的赘瘤需要经过多次的艾灸治疗，才会慢慢脱落，不留一点疤痕。"

秀秀激动地握住鲍姑的手："太谢谢您了，没想到我脸上的赘瘤真的有希望被治好。"

后来，鲍姑又帮秀秀做了几次艾灸治疗。看到秀秀脸上的赘瘤慢慢脱落，越来越美貌，鲍姑心里高兴极了。鲍姑妙手回春，帮助秀秀重拾了信心。在病情痊愈后，秀秀脸上也洋溢起开心的笑容。

鲍姑用灸法治病的事迹还有很多很多，因为她医术高超，深受百姓敬爱，故后人称她治病所用的艾草——采自越秀山山脚下的红脚艾，为"鲍姑艾"。

Bao Gu Treats Disease with Moxibustion

In our daily life, moxibustion is a commonly used means of treating disease and preserving health. Moxibustion therapy has a long history in our country. Since ancient times, doctors have explored and summarized many experiences of moxibustion therapy in medical practice. As what was recorded in history, Bao Gu was the first doctor to treat disease with moxibustion. She liked to study medicine from childhood and was good at pharmacology and moxibustion therapy. The *Record of Bao Gu Temple states*, "Bao Gu treated wart with natural moxa from Yuegang. The wart was removed soon after burning moxa on the diseased part. Many people benefited from this moxibustion method over years." This is the story about Bao Gu treating wart with moxibustion.

In October of one autumn, people were enjoying the the joy of harvest. But in a small village of Yuexiushan mountain, a young girl named Xiu Xiu was very depressed and often cried alone. One day, Xiu Xiu sat alone by the river, looking at her own reflection in the water and muttering sadly, "Why does everyone laugh at me? Shall I never find the ideal husband because of the dark brown warts on my face? I'm so sad. If there were no warts on my face, people would not have laughed at me. Is that right?"

Just then, Bao Gu passed by the river after collecting herbs and heard the crying of Xiuxiu. Bao Gu went to Xiuxiu, handed her a handkerchief, and said, "Don't be sad for other people's words. It's not your fault to suffer from the disease. Anyway, it is not very terrible. I'm a doctor and like to study medicine, Perhaps I can cure the warts on your face." Xiu

Xiu was surprised and said, "Really? Really? Can you really cure the warts on my face?" Bao Gu said, "Yes. Don't be so excited just yet. Let me take a look at your face."

After examining Xiu Xiu carefully, Bao Gu had a solution in her mind. She took out some red-foot wormwood from the medicine bag she carried and said to Xiu Xiu, "Don't worry. I have a method to solve your problem." Bao Gu twisted the red-foot wormwood into moxa wool, lit it, and put it above Xiu Xiu's face. She told Xiu Xiu to inform her if she felt any discomfort. Xiu Xiu whispered a yes and waited in anxiety and anticipation.

After the burning of moxa wool, Bao Gu inspected the warts on Xiuxiu's face carefully and said, "The treatment for this time is over. You need to be treated by moxibustion for many times before the warts can be removed without any scar left." Xiu Xiu held Bao Gu's hands excitedly and said, "Thank you very much. I didn't expect to be cured of the warts on my face, but now it is realized." Later, Bao Gu gave several moxibustion treatments for Xiu Xiu and was happy to see she was becoming beautiful with the warts being removed from her face. With Bao Gu's magic hand, Xiu Xiu was cured and regained confidence, with a happy smile on her face.

There are many stories about Bao Gu treating patients with moxibustion. She was respected and loved by the people for her excellent medical skills.The wormwood she used to treat patients, the red-foot wormwood taken from the foot of Yuexiu Mountain, was called "the Bao Gu wormwood" by later generations.

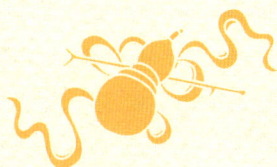

甄权针刺臂痛而复射

提到古代著名的中医医家，很多人都会想到华佗、扁鹊、孙思邈等，他们都是为中医做出极大贡献的人。不过，还有一位与以上医家齐名而立却鲜为人知的医者——甄权。甄权是许州扶沟（今属河南）人，与其兄甄立言皆因母亲患有疾病而学医。后因为医术高超而出名，精通针灸之术，造诣颇深，也熟悉养生之术。据说他活了 103 岁，可见他对于中医治病与养生知识的精通。他一生著述颇多，绘有《明堂人形图》一卷，撰有《针经钞》三卷、《针方》《脉诀

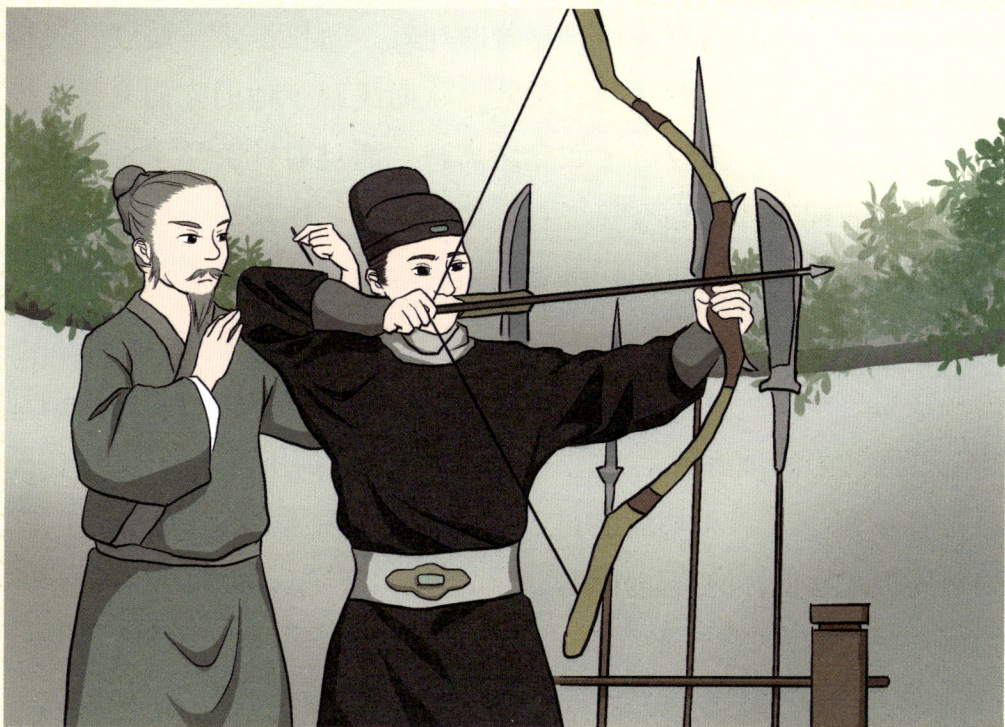

赋》各一卷、《药性论》四卷。他的著作对后世针灸学理论的发展有着深远的影响。下面是一则他诊病的经典案例。

相传隋唐鲁州（今山东）刺史库狄嵚患了风痹证，痛苦不堪，无法拉弓引箭，他请了众多医生医治，但均未奏效。后来，甄权得知后上门仔细诊查病情。和其他医生不一样的是，甄权并没有直接根据病情开汤药，也没有让其在家中好好保养，而是将库狄嵚拉到外边，对他说："你只管拿起弓箭拉弓对准箭靶，我只需要一针你就可以复射。"库狄嵚半信半疑地拉起弓箭，随即甄权瞅准时机，找准穴位，一针刺进他的肩髃穴。就在银针扎进穴位的一瞬间，库狄嵚顿时感到手臂酸胀，一股力量自上臂直冲到手掌，肩膀也不疼了，随即一箭便射中了靶心。众人见状无一不为甄权的医术鼓掌，纷纷称赞他是悬壶济世的神医。

在当时，针灸疗法被广泛应用于治疗各种疾病，因为它不仅没有不良反应，而且具有快速、显著的疗效。甄权也正是通过针灸技术，精准地刺激了库狄嵚的肩髃穴，从而缓解了他的疼痛症状，恢复了手臂的力量。甄权医术如此之高超，而且对针灸学术发展的贡献也很大，那为什么如今很少有人知道他呢？这是因为他的很多著作都失传了，这也是我国针灸界的一大损失，如今只有部分内容可以在孙思邈和王焘的著作中见到，不禁为之惋惜。

最后再来说一下肩髃穴。抬肩时，肩部前后出现两个凹陷的地方，前面凹陷的地方就是此穴位（肩部最高点前下方的凹陷处）。经常按揉肩髃穴，对于肩膀的酸、疼、僵等各种病变有缓解的作用，对肩周炎也有良好的预防作用，一起尝试一下吧。

Zhen Quan Treats Wind Arthralgia with Acupuncture to Make Arrow Shooting Possible Again

When it comes to famous practitioners of Chinese medicine in ancient times, people think of Hua Tuo, Bianque, Sun Simiao, etc. They all have made great contributions to Chinese medicine. Today, however, we are going to tell the story of Zhen Quan, a doctor who is equally famous as the above-mentioned medical experts but less known to most people. Zhen Quan was a native of Fugou, Xu Prefecture (now in Henan Province). He and his brother, Zhen Liyan, both studied medicine to treat the disease of their mother. Later, he became famous for his excellent medical skills and had a good mastery of acupuncture and moxibustion, and the art of health preservation. It is said that he enjoyed a longevity of 103 years, which shows his proficiency in disease treatment and health care. His writings include a volume of *Mingtang Human Figure*, three volumes of *Collected Writings of Acupuncture Classics*, one volume of *Acupuncture Formulas*, one volume of *Pulse Diagnosis Technique*, and four volumes of *Treatise on Medicinal Properties*. These writings had a profound influence on the development and formation of Chinese acupuncture theory in later times. The following is the classic case of his medical diagnosis.

According to legend, She Diqin, the prefectural governor of Lu Zhou (now Shandong province) in the Sui and Tang Dynasty, was suffering from migratory arthralgia with symptoms of unbearable pain and inability to shoot arrow. He invited many doctors to treat the disease but in vain. Later, Zhen Quan came to his home after learning his condition and examined him carefully. Unlike other doctors, Zhen Quan did not prescribe medicine directly, nor ask him to take care of health at home, but took She Diqin outside and said to him, "Just pick up your bow and arrow, and direct at the target. I would treat with one needle, and you could be able to shoot again." She Diqin drew the bow and arrow doubtfully, then Zhen Quan located the acupoint and needled his Jianyu acupoint at the right moment. When the silver needle probed into the acupoint, She Diqin felt sore and swollen in the arm immediately. A force rushed from the upper arm straight to the palm, his shoulder pain vanished and he hit the center of the target. The crowd applauded for Zhen Quan's medical skill and praised him as a highly-skilled doctor who could help people around the world.

At that time, acupuncture therapy was widely used to treat various diseases because it not only had no side effects, but also had fast and effective healing effects. It was through the technique of acupuncture that Zhen Quan precisely stimulated the Jianyu acupoint (LI 15) of She Diqin, thus relieving his pain and restoring the strength of his arm. Why is Zhen Quan, who was so skilled in medical field and contributed so much to the academic development of acupuncture, relatively unknown today? The reason is that many of his writings have been lost, which is a great loss to the acupuncture circle in China. Today, only part of his writings can be seen in the books of Sun Simiao and Wang Tao, which is truely regrettable.

Finally, let's talk about the Jianyu acupoint (LI 15). When we lift our shoulders, there are two sunken places in the front and back respectively. The one in the front is Jianyu acupoint (the front inner point below the highest point of the shoulder). Whenever we have problems of shoulder pain and stiff neck, we can press and knead the Jianyu acupoint to relieve the symptoms and prevent periarthritis of the shoulders. Let's try it together!

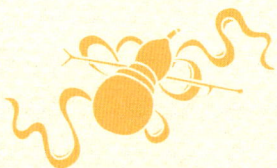

孙思邈治疗唐太宗李世民

　　孙思邈，唐代著名的医药学家，被后人尊称为"药王"。他医术高超、医德高尚，集毕生治病经验著成对后世影响深远的医学巨著《备急千金要方》《千金翼方》。

　　唐太宗李世民年轻的时候封号是秦王，他曾受命于父亲李渊，去攻打驻守在天水城的薛举。李世民急于打胜仗立功，攻城计划准备不够完善，多次攻城后，不仅没有成功，而且军队损失惨重。随着一次一次的失败，军心越来越动摇。李世民看到此情此景，心中忧虑无比，最终病倒在军营里。

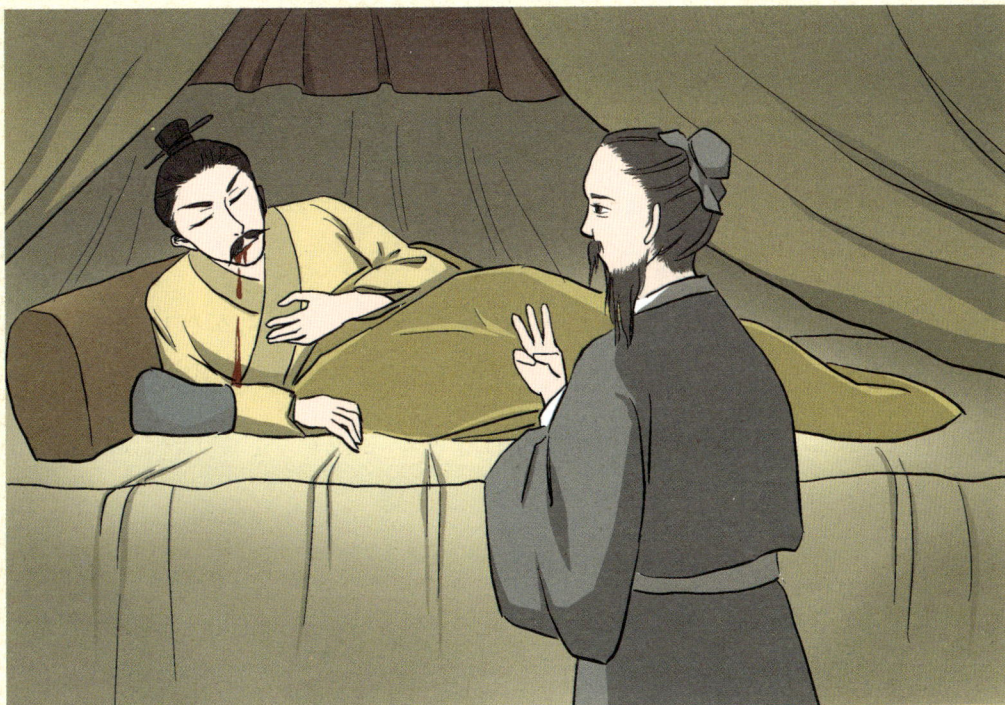

李渊听到儿子的病讯，十分担忧，连夜派了几名御医从京城出发，前去为李世民治病。御医们挨个给李世民诊脉，一致认为李世民的病主要是肝火郁结、忧思太过导致的。但是，李世民喝了几日汤药后，病情却没有丝毫好转。

军师看在眼里，急在心里，就悄悄去问御医是何缘故。御医无奈，答道："秦王身份尊贵，我们开方子要小心谨慎，不能用太猛的药，只能用一些温和的药，效果自然就大打折扣。"

此时，恰巧孙思邈听说了这件事，就去军营自荐，说自己可以试试。军师连忙将孙思邈请进来，孙思邈诊脉后，把军师拉到一边，说道："现在秦王的病情，用一般的汤药和针石之术只治标不治本，我会说一些话激怒秦王，怒火攻心时扎针，能够帮助他把瘀血排出来，一会儿还需要麻烦军师帮我解释。"军师说："只要能治好秦王的病，让我做什么都可以。"孙思邈听闻此言，小声对军师交代："一会儿不管我说什么，军师都不要当真。"

于是，孙思邈来到秦王的病床前，取出银针，做欲治疗状。他对秦王说："最近有多位御医为殿下诊治，都没有效果，殿下应该明白，目前找不到能医治好殿下的大夫了。我能够治好殿下，但是我要提三个条件，殿下答应了我，我才肯施治。"

李世民虚弱地躺在床上，心中颇为不快，心想这人也太过狂妄了！却只能无奈道："你说说看，只要我能做到，我就答应你。"

孙思邈说："如果我把您的病治好了，我第一个条件就是要您身上的这身衣袍。"

李世民说："这有何妨，拿去便是！"

孙思邈继续道："第二个条件就是我想从您的妻妾中挑一位合心意的，您把她赏赐给我，怎么样？"

李世民怒目而视："你好大的胆子，居然敢觊觎我的妻妾。"

孙思邈说："对，听闻殿下的妻妾貌美贤惠，我有意得之。"

李世民心中极为愤怒，却不得不强忍怒气，说："好，好，好！我答应你，第三个条件是什么？"

孙思邈哈哈大笑，说："殿下果然大方，我最后一个条件就是让这李唐天下姓孙！"

李世民听后气得火冒三丈，双目瞪视，满面赤红。孙思邈见此情形，立刻将银针刺入他心肺间瘀血处。李世民随即吐出大口黑血，顿感身心舒畅，体内的瘀血已顺利排出。

事后，军师给李世民讲明孙思邈故意出言不逊的缘由。李世民不但没有怪罪孙思邈，还大赞他的医术、才智和胆识，并想给他封官进爵。但孙思邈拒绝了李世民的嘉奖，继续云游四海，在民间救治百姓。

Sun Simiao Treated the Disease of Li Shimin, Emperor Taizong of Tang Dynasty

Sun Simiao, a famous medical pharmacist in the Tang Dynasty, was honored as the "King of Medicine" by later generations. With his excellent medical skills and noble medical ethics, he summarized his clinical experience in disease treatment and compiled *Beiji Qianjin Yao Fang* and *Qianjin Yi Fang*, which had a great influence for later generations.

When Li Shimin, Emperor Taizong of Tang, was young, he was titled King of Qin and ordered by his father Li Yuan to attack Xue Ju, who was stationed in the city of Tianshui. Eager to win the battle for meritorious service, Li Shimin did not prepare enough before the attack. After many trials, he failed and his troops suffered heavy loss. With one failure after another, the morale of the army wavered. Facing this situation, Li Shimin was very worried and fell ill in the barracks eventually.

When Li Yuan heard his son's illness, he was anxious and sent several imperial physicians from the capital overnight to treat Li Shimin. The imperial physicians took pulse for Li Shimin one by one and drew the same conclusion that the disease of Li Shimin was mainly caused by stagnation of liver fire and excessive worry. However, Li Shimin did not improve after taking decoctions for a few days.

Seeing this, the military counsellor was anxious and went to the imperial physicians for the reason. The imperial physicians replied in helplessness, "Considering the distinguished identity of the King of Qin, we were very cautious in prescribing medicinal herbs. We could only prescribe herbs with mild property instead of those with strong property, which would influence the curative effect naturally."

At this time, Sun Simiao happened to hear about this matter, and went to the military camp to recommend himself for the treatment. The military counsellor immediately invited Sun Simiao in. After examining the pulse of Li Shimin, Sun Simiao pulled the military counsellor aside and said, "Now the disease of the King of Qin was very severe, and the ordinary decoctions and needling method could only serve as temporary solutions instead of curative ones. I will say something to irritate the King of Qin and then give acupuncture treatment when he is angry to help remove his static blood. I need your help later to explain this for me." The military counsellor said, "I will do anything as long as it can cure the disease of the King of Qin." Sun Simiao whispered to him, "No matter what I say later, do not take it seriously."

Then Sun Simiao came to the bed of the King of Qin and took out the silver needles, as if he would treat with acupuncture. He said to the King of Qin, "Recently, many imperial physicians have tried to treat disease for you but in vain. You should be clear that presently, there is no other doctor but me who can cure your disease. But before that, I have three conditions for you to help meet. Otherwise, I will not carry out the treatment."

Lying on the bed weakly, Li Shimin felt very unhappy about Sun Simiao's conceitedness. He said unwillingly, "Tell me your conditions. I will agree if I am capable of meeting them."

Sun Simiao said, "If I can cure your disease, I want the set of clothes on your body."

Li Shimin said, "What does it matter? Take it if you like!"

Sun Simiao continued, "If I can cure your disease, my second condition is to select one of your wives and concubines I like. You need to give her to me. How about that?"

Li Shimin glared, "How dare you covet my wives and concubines!"

Sun Simiao said, "Yes, Your Highness. I have heard that they are very beautiful and virtuous, and I am inclined to have one of them."

Being mad in heart, Li Shimin had to restrain his anger and said, "Well, well, well! I agree. What's the third condition?"

Sun Simiao laughed loudly and said, "Your Highness is really generous. My last condition is that the Tang Dynasty ruled by your Li family now will be ruled by my Sun family!"

After hearing this, Li Shimin became extremely furious with glaring eyes and a red face. At this time, Sun Simiao inserted silver needles into the stagnated place between his heart and lung at once. Then Li Shimin spit out a mouthful of black blood and felt comfortable and pleasant immediately. The static blood in his body had been expelled successfully.

Afterwards, the military counsellor explained to Li Shimin about the reason for Sun Simiao's rude remarks. Li Shimin did not blame Sun Simiao. On the contrary, he praised Sun Simiao for his superb medical skill, his wisdom and his courage, and wanted to offer official post for Sun Simiao. But Sun Simiao refused his offer and continued his travel around the world, treating and curing diseases for the people with his medical skills.

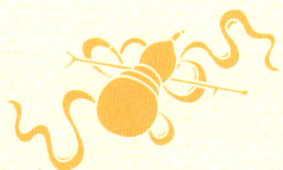

甄权针灸著作影响唐代刑罚

甄权，唐代著名针灸医家，许州扶沟人，每每给患者治疗都能针到病除。李世民当亲王时讨伐过王世充，任命李袭誉为潞州总管。李袭誉的随军医生中就有甄权，但是当时甄权的名气还不是很大。甄权发现当时的医生多注重用中药治疗疾病，忽视了针灸的重要性，于是他结合所学画成了《明堂人形图》。该图主要讲述人体的穴位和针灸操作，也被称为《明堂针灸图》。甄权把这幅图交给了李袭誉，但李袭誉并没有当回事。后来李世民继位当皇帝后，李袭誉入朝为官。此时，甄权已经不在李袭誉身边了，但他在民间四处行医，声誉日渐隆

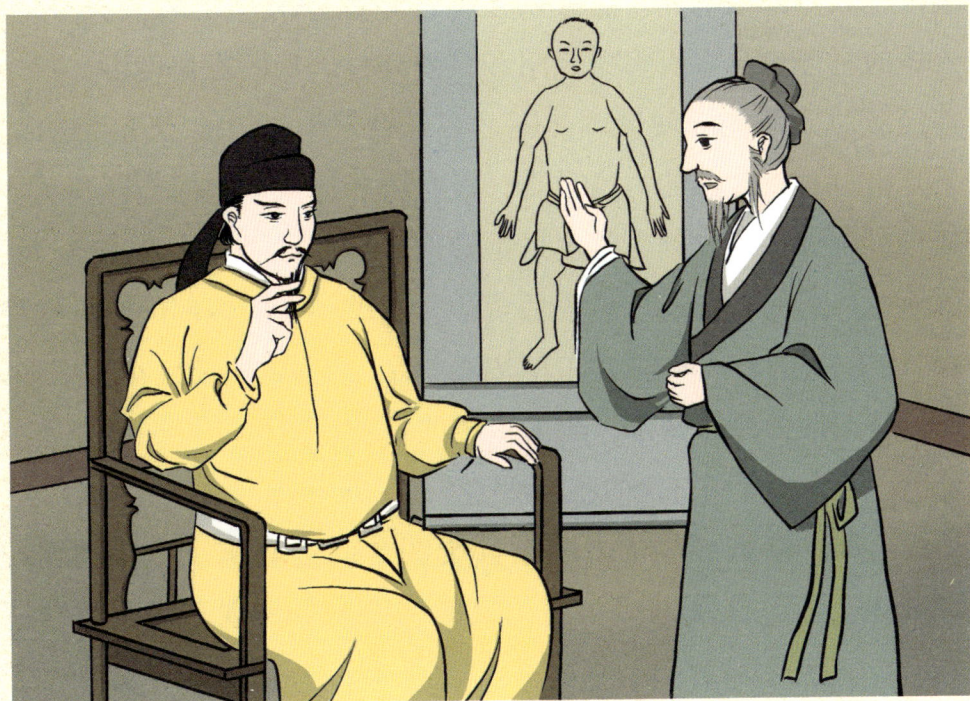

盛。李袭誉颇有耳闻，这才想起来当初甄权献给他的《明堂针灸图》，并向唐太宗李世民大大地称赞了这幅图的精妙之处。

唐太宗是个开明的君主，喜欢招贤纳士，他非常重视甄权的《明堂针灸图》。出于对甄权高明医术的肯定，唐太宗特地请来甄权对《明堂针灸图》进行仔细的修订和完善。不久，修订好的官方版《明堂针灸图》就问世了。这幅画制作精美，图文并茂。唐太宗见到后，连连称赞，在研究欣赏之际，还下诏修改了当时的一项刑法。

唐代所使用的五刑之法包括笞、杖、徒、流、死五等。其中笞刑是指用竹板或荆条鞭打犯人的背部，是最轻的刑罚，但是由于实施刑罚的人下手轻重不同，打死的人并不少，相反更重的徒刑、流放却会少死很多人。唐太宗继位以来，为了开创盛世，在刑罚方面一直是力求宽大仁慈。甄权性情仁厚，当初决定学医，就是想要救治自己病重的母亲。甄权出于对犯人的同情，向唐太宗建议应当取消鞭打犯人背部的刑罚。唐太宗在看过《明堂针灸图》之后，才发现人体的背部也分布有多条经络和重要穴位。从医家角度讲，很多背部经脉腧穴不能随便针刺，施针时一针不慎，可能会伤及性命。如果是鞭打犯人背部的力度过重，极有可能造成严重内伤，甚至导致死亡。唐太宗意识到，笞刑虽是轻刑，但却可能会使人丧命，于是就下令以后的笞刑不许打人后背。又考虑到人的臀部肉厚，经络又少，用同样的力气和刑具打人臀部的话，致死的可能性小了很多。因此，笞刑改为鞭笞臀部。唐太宗更改笞刑，减少了行刑后犯人的意外伤亡。许多受到笞刑的犯人活了下来，拥有改过自新的机会。

就这样，甄权绘制的《明堂针灸图》间接影响了唐代刑罚的故事成为美谈。这既说明了唐太宗的仁政，也体现了医家的慈悲之心。

The Influence of Zhen Quan's Acupuncture and Moxibustion Works on the Penalty of the Tang Dynasty

Zhen Quan, a native of Fugou, Xuzhou, was a well-known acupuncturist in the Tang Dynasty, who could always cure diseases with needling method. As a prince, Li Shimin once appointed Li Xiyu as the governor of Luzhou when he was suppressing Wang Shichong. Zhen Quan was among Li Xiyu's military doctors then, but not very famous. Zhen Quan found that doctors at that time stressed the usage of medicinal herbs to treat diseases but neglected the importance of acupuncture. So he drew the *Human Figure Diagram of Ming Hall* to illustrate the acupoints and acupuncture manipulation techniques. It was also known as the *Acupuncture Diagram of Ming Tang*. Zhen Quan gave this diagram to Li Xiyu, but he did not take it seriously. Later, Li Shimin succeeded to the throne and Li Xiyu became an official in the imperial court. At this time, Zhen Quan was not with Li Xiyu anymore and practiced medicine among the people with growing reputation. Li Xiyu heard about Zhen Quan and recalled the *Acupuncture Diagram of Ming Tang* given to him by Zhen Quan. So Li Xiyu gave the diagram to Li Shimin (Emperor Taizong of Tang Dynasty) and praised it greatly.

Emperor Taizong of Tang was an enlightened monarch who liked to recruit virtuous talents. He attached great importance to Zhen Quan's *Acupuncture Diagram of Ming Tang* and affirmed his superb medical skills. Then Emperor Taizong of Tang invited Zhen Quan to revise and improve the diagram carefully and issued the revised official version of this diagram, which was exquisitely and beautifully illustrated. While appreciating the diagram, Emperor Taizong of Tang issued an imperial edict to revise a penalty.

In the Tang Dynasty, the five forms of punishment were flogging, caning, imprisonment, exile, and death penalty. Among them, flogging was the lightest form of punishment, which was to whip the prisoner on the back with a bamboo board or a twig of the chaste tree. Although it seemed to be the lightest punishment, it could lead to more deaths due to the different degree of severity in the process of carrying out the punishment than other forms of punishment like imprisonment and exile. Since the reign of Emperor Taizong of Tang, he has always strove to be lenient and merciful in terms of punishment to create a prosperous nation. Zhen Quan was good natured and decided to study medicine originally with the purpose to save his mother. Therefore, out of sympathy for the prisoners, Zhen Quan suggested to Emperor Taizong of Tang that the punishment of whipping the prisoners on the back should be abolished. After reading the *Acupuncture Diagram of Ming Tang* , Emperor Taizong of Tang found that there were many meridians and acupoints on the back of the human body, which should be needled cautiously when being selected for acupuncture treatment, and otherwise might lead to death. If the prisoners were whipped severely on the back, they might suffer from internal damage even death. Emperor Taizong of Tang realized that flogging, though as a light punishment, could also kill people, which was very unreasonable. He ordered that in the future, flogging was forbidden to be carried out by whipping the back of people. Considering that the buttock part was thick with flesh and few with meridians, the whipping on the buttock would cause less deaths if the same strength and instruments were used.

Thus, flogging on the back was changed to flogging on the buttock by Emperor Taizong of Tang, which reduced many unexpected deaths after the penalties. This made it possible for the prisoners who were punished by flogging to survive and make a fresh start.

This is the much-told story about the *Acupuncture Diagram of Ming Tang* drawn by Zhen Quan indirectly affecting the penalty of the Tang Dynasty. It not only indicates the benevolent reign of Emperor Taizong of Tang, but also reflects the compassionate heart of the doctors.

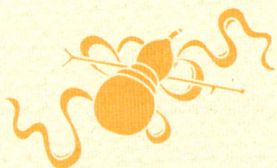

秦鸣鹤刺穴放血治唐高宗头风

　　唐代著名中医药学家孙思邈曾经说过："胆欲大而心欲小，智欲圆而行欲方。"这句话表明医生在行医时应该胆大心细。可是如果时逢皇上重病，医生敢不敢诊治呢？要知道当时医生的地位很低，稍有差错或者言语不当就会带来杀身之祸。但是有一位医生却做到了胆大心细，勇敢自信，他就是和孙思邈同时代的名医秦鸣鹤。他论医术不输孙思邈，论胆魄不输华佗，他刺穴放血治唐高宗头风的故事同样流传至今。

　　丙戌年（公元 626 年）十一月，唐高宗李治旧疾发作，头部沉重疼痛难忍，眼睛昏花，不能视物，苦不堪言。此病是皇帝的老顽

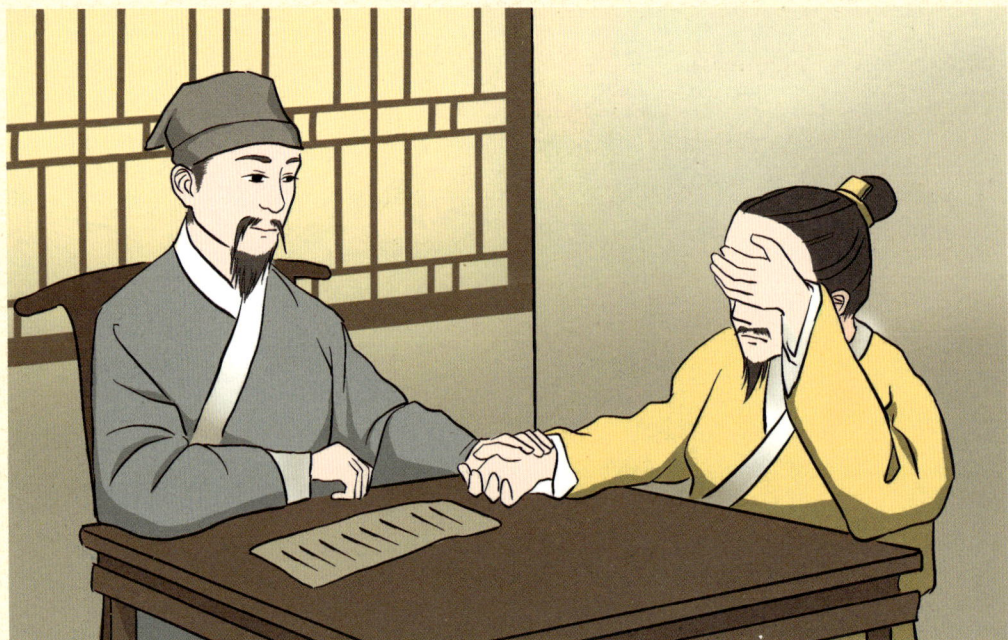

疾，很多太医都束手无策，也没人敢站出来为他医治，害怕稍有闪失便祸及自身。这时，秦鸣鹤站了出来，说他可以为皇上医治，顿时哗然四起。但秦鸣鹤没有因此而受到影响。起身上前观察病情后，他告诉皇上这个病叫"头风"，恳请用针刺头部穴位放血，这样才能够治愈此疾病。这时候整个朝堂鸦雀无声，没人敢发言，也许正在心里暗暗讨论秦鸣鹤，想看他的笑话。正在大家不知所措之时，皇后武则天愤怒地说："把他拖下去斩了，竟想在皇帝头上放血，真是大逆不道。"秦鸣鹤没有因此而胆怯，而是跪在地上等待唐高宗的命令。皇上说："没事，朕得此病久矣，疼痛难忍，不治必死，让他来为我治疗吧，未必效果不好。"听到命令后，秦鸣鹤小心地走上前，用针具点刺百会、脑户穴放血。片刻之后，唐高宗感觉耳聪目明，神清气爽。不仅当面赞赏了秦鸣鹤，还给予他很多银子和布匹，就连武则天见状也觉得刚才有失妥当，随即表示歉意。就这样，秦鸣鹤在长安城顿时名声大噪，他为皇帝治病的故事也在民间流传开来。

　　秦鸣鹤刺穴放血治愈唐高宗头风的佳话，启示医者应具备高度的职业道德和责任心，要注重细节和技巧的应用。学子们亦应如是，心怀自信，坚信已有所长，切勿轻视自我。当机遇降临，更要毫不犹豫地紧抓机遇，毋忧失败之虑。宝剑锻炼十年方可成，信心与付出终将换来未来辉煌的成就。

Qin Minghe Treats the Head Wind of Emperor Tang Gaozong with Acupuncture Bloodletting

Sun Simiao, a famous Chinese medical expert in the Tang Dynasty, once said, "The courage is to be big and the heart is to be small, the wisdom is to be round and the behavior is to be square." This is to remind doctors should be bold and careful in the medical practice. However, if the emperor was seriously ill, did you dare to treat him as a doctor? The status of doctor at that time was very low, the slightest mistake or improper words would bring fatal disaster. Nevertheless, there was a doctor who was bold, cautious, brave and confident. His name is Qin Minghe, a famous doctor living contemporarily with Sun Simiao. His medical skill and boldness are not inferior to Sun Simiao and Hua Tuo. Let us look at the story of Qin Minghe's treating the head wind of Emperor Tang Gaozong with acupuncture bloodletting methods.

In November of the year Bingwu (626 AD), Emperor Gaozong of Tang (Li Zhi) suffered from chronic disease again unspeakably with symptoms of severe headache and blurred vision. This disease, being the emperor's recurring disease, was hard to treat and no palace physician dared to stand out for the treatment with the fear of possible disaster. At this time, Qin Minghe came forward and said he wanted to have a try to treat the emperor, which caused an uproar. Qin Minghe was not affected by this and began to diagnose the emperor. He told the emperor that the disease was called "head wind" and could be treated with bloodletting by needling acupoints on the head. Hearing this, all people at the court was silent and no one dared to speak, perhaps secretly thinking that Qin Minghe would become a joke. All being at a loss. Empress Wu Zetian said angrily, "Drag him down and behead him. How dare you let blood on the head of the emperor? This is monstrous crime." Qin Minghe knelt down to wait for the order of Emperor Gaozong of Tang without any cowardliness. The emperor said, "It's okay. I've suffered from this disease for a long time with unbearable pains. I would die without timely treatment. Let him have a try and the result might not be bad." So Qin Minghe stepped forward carefully and needled the "Baihui acupoint (GV 20)" and "Naohu acupoint (GV 17)" to let blood. A few moments later, Emperor Gaozong of Tang felt better with normal hearing and clear eyesight and refreshed spirit and mind. He praised Qin Minghe directly and gave him a lot of money and cloths as awards. Wu Zetian also apologized for her improper words before. In this way, Qin Minghe became famous in Chang'an City and the story of his treating disease for the emperor spread among the people.

The above story serves as good inspiration for doctors to possess a high degree of professional ethics and responsibility, and to adhere importance to details and application of medical skills. As students, we should be confident about our own strengths and never underestimate ourselves. When the opportunity comes, we should seize it unhesitatingly and be free from the fear of failure. Just as the sword that must be forged for ten years to turn to a treasured blade, marvelous success in the future could only be achieved by great confidence and efforts.

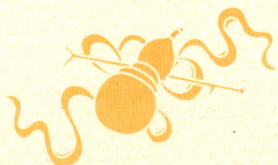

王惟一铸造天圣针灸铜人

　　王惟一是北宋名医，担任过两朝医官，在医学尤其是针灸上造诣深厚，同时在金石雕刻方面也颇有研究。王惟一发现针灸教学使用的针灸图谱过于单一，不够生动形象，而且还有错误，不但教学不方便，还容易误人子弟，伤人害命。于是王惟一产生了设计制作准确无误又立体形象的针灸人体模型的想法。当时他曾两次向皇帝提出要铸造针灸铜人的请求，宋仁宗以为："古经训诂至精，学者执封多失，传心岂如会目，著辞不若案形，复令创铸铜人为式。"在朝廷批准之后，王惟一负责设计，朝廷负责组织工匠，于天圣五年，

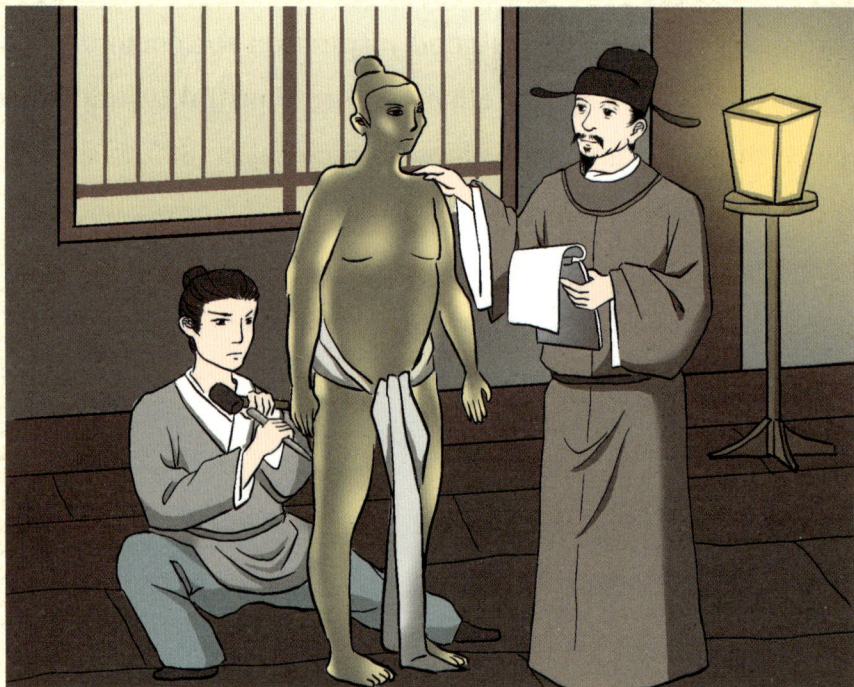

两座针灸铜人模型铸造成功。宋仁宗非常满意，将其中一座放在翰林医官院用来针灸教学，另一座放在大相国寺仁济殿以供百姓观摩。

宋天圣针灸铜人是与真人等大的裸体男像，用精铜铸造而成。铜人表面刻有手三阳经、手三阴经、足三阳经、足三阴经与任督两脉共 14 条经脉的循行路线及 354 个腧穴的位置，均严格按照人体的实际比例刻制，并且体内雕有脏腑，位置、大小、形态与真人基本符合，此后一直被奉为"国宝"。起先，王惟一铸造针灸铜人时就是想将其应用于教学，但是如何能知道穴位找得准不准呢？他用蜡将穴位都封起来，里面装满水银，如果扎到准确位置，就会有水银流出来，反之就没有水银流出来。为了让铜人里的水银能够源源不断地流出来，他就把模型做成双层，再分成上下两个部分，夹层里可以注水银，并且在发髻处做一个注入水银的装置。这样的构造可以使天圣针灸铜人的穴孔与身体内部相通，在考核和教学时，如果针刺部位不准确、针刺角度与深度不合适，针具就不能刺入铜人体内，只有将针具刺入准确的部位、适当的角度和深度，才能恰好扎在被堵的穴孔上，针具就能刺到体腔内，拔出针后，水银就能从穴孔处流出。这种使用实物模型的方式是形象教学方法的重大突破。天圣针灸铜人是世界上第一座描绘了人体经脉、经穴的模型，也是世界上第一座展示了人体骨骼、内脏的模型，开创了医学模型考试的先河。

宋天圣针灸铜人设计精巧无比，制作出神入化。它的成功铸造是医学史上的一大创举，无论是在我国还是在世界都引起了极大关注。它的问世，既体现了当时劳动人民令人赞叹的人体美学艺术，又表现了我国古人精湛的铸造水平。时至今日，针灸铜人模型依然具有很高的学习和研究价值。

Wang Weiyi Forged Bronze Acupuncture Figure during Tiansheng Period

Wang Weiyi (987—1067AD), a famous doctor in the Northern Song Dynasty, served as a medical official in the Emperor Renzong and the Emperor Yingzong of the Song dynasties. He was very accomplished in medicine, especially acupuncture and moxibustion, and in metal and stone carving as well. Wang Weiyi found that the acupuncture and moxibustion mapping used in medical education was not comprehensive and vivid enough, even with mistakes. This was very inconvenient for teaching and might let young people stray from the right path or cause injury and death. Thus, Wang Weiyi decided to design and forge an accurate and three-dimensional acupuncture mannequin. He put forward this suggestion to the Emperor Renzong of Song Dynasty twice. The emperor responded, "The explanation of words in ancient classic books was exquisite, but some were lost due to the inflexibility of the scholars. To have a direct look is better than understanding with imagination, and to create a substantial form is better than explaining with words. The bronze acupuncture figure is permitted to be forged." With the approval from the imperial court, Wang Weiyi designed and forged two bronze acupuncture figures in the fifth year of Tiansheng period with the help of some craftsmen. The emperor was very satisfied and ordered to place one in the Hanlin Medical Academy for teaching purpose and the other in the Renji Hall of the Daxiangguo Temple for imperial inspection.

This bronze acupuncture figure is a life-size nude male figure forged with fine copper. On the surface of the bronze figure, there are circulation routes of the 14 meridians, namely the three yang meridians of hand, the three yin meridians of hand, the three yang meridians of foot, the three yin meridians of foot, the Conception vessel and Governor vessel, and 354 acupoints. The meridians and acupoints and the viscera were all carved in strict accordance with the actual proportion, location and size of the real human body. The internal structure of the figure was also exquisitely constructed. Since then, it has been regarded as a "national treasure" in successive dynasties. The original goal for Wang Weiyi to forge this bronze figure is to teach acupuncture, but a question arose: How to know that the acupoint was accurately located? Then he came up with the idea of filling the bronze figure with mercury and sealing all the acupoints with wax. If the acupoint was located and needled accurately, mercury would flow out of the bronze figure, otherwise it would not. To enable the continuous flowing of mercury, he made the bronze figure double-layered and divided it into upper and lower parts. Water could be contained in the interlayer space and poured in from the bun of the figure with a device. Such structure could make the acupoints connected with the internal parts of the bronze figure. During medical examination and teaching, water or mercury was poured into the bronze figure. If the location, the needling angle and depth were not correctly manipulated, the needling instruments would not prick into the bronze figure. If they were correctly manipulated, the needling instruments would be inserted into the right acupoint, and water or mercury would flow out when they were withdrawn. This application of physical model in teaching was a crucial breakthrough of image teaching. In the history of medicine, the acupuncture bronze figure of Tiansheng period is the world's first physical model depicting the meridians and acupoints of the human body. It is also the world's first model displaying the human skeleton and viscera, which creates the first form of medical examination with physical models.

The acupuncture bronze figure of Tiansheng period is exquisitely designed and produced, serving as a great innovation in the medical history and attracting attention from both domestic and abroad. It is a vivid reflection of the working people's amazing aesthetic art of human body and the ancient people's exquisite forging skill. Up to now, the bronze acupuncture figure is still of high value for medical study and research.

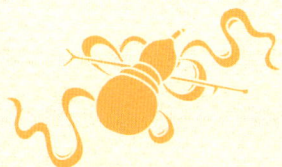

灸法治好背疮

　　中医是中国优秀传统文化的瑰宝，而针灸作为中医的特色疗法之一，在诊治疾病时有很好的疗效。古典医籍中记载的诸多医案，可以帮助人们很好地认识针灸。比如，《医说》中就记载了一则灸法治疗背疮的故事。

　　故事发生在北宋的都城开封府。一日，家住万胜门的王超忽然感觉身体不适，背上似乎长了疮疡，疼痛难忍，他赶忙找到一家医馆请大夫医治。大夫解开王超的衣服，看到背上的疮疡已经如灯盏般大小，疮头遍布。叹息道："你的背疮很严重啊！需要赶紧治疗，我建议你去梁门里，外科金龟儿张家的大夫能治疗你的背疮。"王超连忙道谢，去梁门里的路上心中忐忑，希望张大夫能有办法治好自

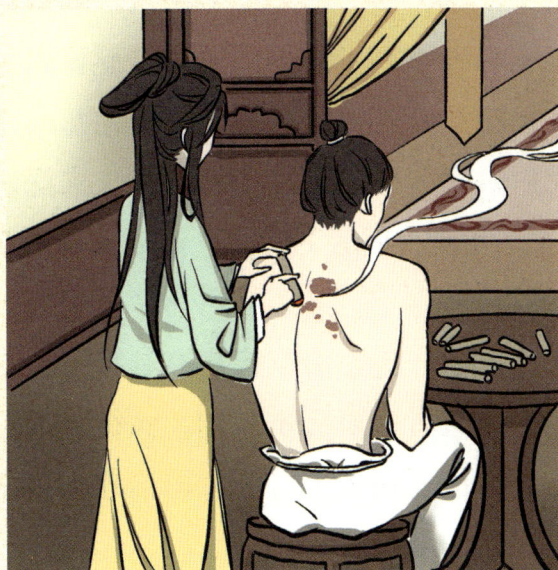

己的背疮。

到了张家医馆后，张大夫仔细诊察王超的病情，频频皱眉，对他说："你的背疮很严重，不是中药所能治疗的。只有采用艾灸的方法，或许有希望能治好你的病，然而治疗过程也会颇为费力。"王超说："张大夫，只要有希望能治好我的背疮，我愿意一试。"于是，张大夫吩咐徒弟制作了一些艾条，让王超带回家，叮嘱他："你回家后，让家人帮你在背疮上做艾灸治疗，刚开始艾灸的时候，你可能感觉不到疼痛，要继续灸下去，直到感到疼痛的时候，灸量才足以达到治疗的效果。记住，一定要灸到感觉疼痛了才可以结束治疗。等艾灸完之后再来复诊。"

回家后，家人按照张大夫的方法为王超做艾灸。艾灸十余壮后，王超还没有感觉到疼痛。妻子焦急地哭了起来，王超安慰妻子道："不要担心，应该是艾灸的量还不够，还没有达到能治疗我背疮的有效刺激量，再继续灸吧。"等到艾灸十三壮的时候，王超"哎呦"一声，艾灸的部位剧烈疼痛起来，背疮旁边腐败的疮肉经过艾灸后都翻卷起来，用手一碰，都掉落在地上，很快长疮的部位就有稍稍愈合的迹象。王超和妻子对张大夫的医术深感佩服。第二天再去复诊，张大夫给了王超几副外敷的药贴，嘱咐他每日将药贴外敷在背疮上，坚持用完后，就能痊愈了。王超对张大夫深表谢意，张大夫笑道："治病救人是我作为医者的责任，看到你的背疮能治好，我也很高兴。"

这个医案告诉人们，艾灸治疗疾病有其独特的疗效，而且灸量是治病的关键。作为医者，要医术高明，医德高尚；作为患者，要有治愈疾病的信心，也要积极配合医生的治疗方案，才能达到最佳的治疗效果。

The Treatment of Sores on the Back with Moxibustion

Traditional Chinese medicine is the treasure of traditional Chinese culture. As a particular therapy, acupuncture and moxibustion can be used to treat diseases effectively. Many medical cases recorded in ancient Chinese medical literature can help us better understand acupuncture and moxibustion. For example, a story about the treatment of sores on the back by moxibustion was recorded in the *History of Medical Schools.*

The story took place in Kaifeng Prefecture in the Northern Song Dynasty. One day, Wang Chao, a person lived in Wanshengmen, suddenly felt sick and suffered from unbearable pain on the back like that caused by sores. He rushed to a doctor, and after taking down his coat, the doctor saw lamp-sized sores on his back. The doctor said, " The sores on your back are very serious. You need urgent treatment. I suggest you go to Liangmen to seek help from doctor Zhang, who is from a medical family known for surgery." Wang Chao thanked the doctor and hurried to Liangmen, being anxious on the way and hoping to be cured by doctor Zhang.

When Wang Chao arrived at the hospital of Zhang family, he was examined by doctor Zhang carefully. Doctor Zhang frowned frequently and said to him, "The sores on your back are very serious and can't be cured with medicinal herbs. Moxibustion can be tried with the hope of treating your disease, though with some efforts." Wang Chao said, "I am willing to try it as long as there is hope of curing the sores on my back." So doctor Zhang told his apprentice to make some moxa sticks for Wang Chao to take home. He told Wang Chao, "When you go home, ask your family member to carry out moxibustion treatment on your back. You may not feel painful at the beginning. Keep on, and the curative effect can only be achieved when you feel painful. Remember, the moxibustion can only be ended until you feel painful. After the moxibustion treatment, come back to me again."

After returning home, the family member carried out moxibustion for Wang Chao according to doctor Zhang's instruction. After burning ten moxa cones, Wang Chao did not feel any pain. His wife cried out of anxiety. Wang Chao comforted her and said, "Don't worry. It might because the amount of moxibustion is not enough to simulate the sores on my back. Let's continue." When burning the thirteenth moxa cones, Wang Chao gave an "ouch" and felt great pain at the diseased region. The rotten flesh near the sores rolled up and fell down on the ground when touched with hand. Soon the diseased part showed sign of healing. Wang Chao and his wife were deeply impressed by doctor Zhang's medical skill. The next day, they went to doctor Zhang again, and he gave Wang Chao several transdermal patches for daily external application on the back. He told Wang Chao he would be cured when the patches were used up. Wang Chao thanked doctor Zhang deeply. Doctor Zhang smiled and said, "It is my duty as a doctor to cure diseases and save people. I am also very happy that the sores on your back could be cured."

This medical case tells us that moxibustion has its unique curative effect in treating diseases, and the amount of it is the key to the effect. As a doctor, one needs to improve medical skills and possess noble medical ethics. As a patient, one needs to have confidence to cure the disease and cooperate actively with the doctor to achieve the best treatment effect.

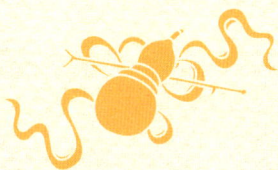

王执中灸治鼻出血

　　相信大家都有过鼻出血的经历，除外伤导致鼻出血外，其他情况的鼻出血或多或少都反映了身体的问题。鼻出血时，应及时采取措施止血。可轻轻用手捏住鼻翼，让血液凝固，同时头部尽量向前，避免咽下血液刺激胃肠道。如果鼻出血持续时间较长或者频繁发生，建议及时就医。医生通过细致的检查找出出血的原因，并制定相应的治疗方案。鼻出血的中医名称叫"鼻衄"，那么在古代人们是怎样治疗鼻出血的呢？下面是古代名医王执中治疗鼻出血的故事。

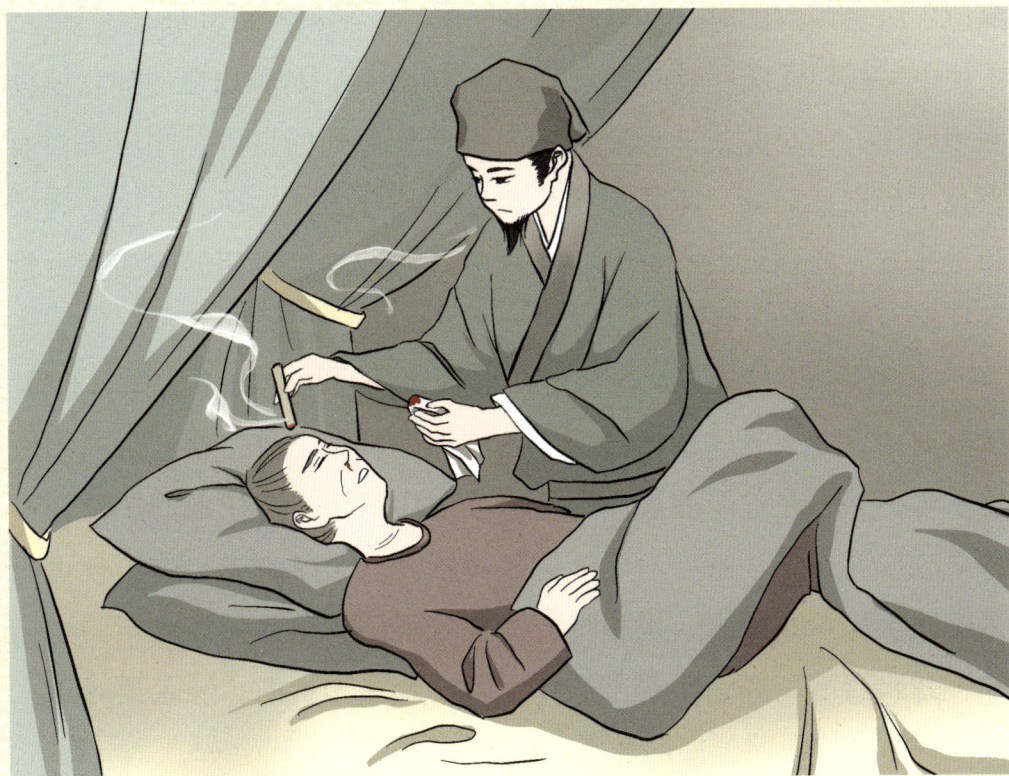

　　王执中，字叔权，南宋时期著名的针灸医药学家。有一天，他母亲忽然鼻出血不止，作为医生的王执中根据自己的经验，赶紧给母亲抓药施治，本以为药到病除，效如桴鼓，但结果让王执中大吃一惊，服用方药过后母亲的鼻出血症状并没有减轻，平时给他人服用且疗效很好的方子都对他母亲无效。此时王执中非常着急，急忙翻看医书，寻找其他治疗此病的方法，希望可以尽快解除母亲的痛苦。当翻阅众多书籍后，他看到《集效方》中说："嘴中和鼻中出血不止的病叫脑衄，可在上星穴位上施灸50壮。"一开始王执中看到施灸50壮时还怀疑这本书的可信性，因为根据经验头部穴位多数不能施行灸法，但此时也没有其他更好的办法治疗，便只能先按书上的方法施治。考虑到治疗过程中的安全性，王执中一开始很谨慎，只灸了7壮。结果疗效很好，母亲鼻子不再流血，王执中大喜，深感中医奥妙的同时，也将此法牢记于心。不料次日其母鼻衄复发，王执中又按照此法在其头部穴位灸了14壮后，鼻腔出血的症状就彻底治好了，未再复发。因此案例习得治疗鼻衄的良方，此后每当有人鼻子出血的时候，王执中都会教他们治疗方法，即灸头部的囟会和上星穴，此病就会有好转直至痊愈。这种治疗鼻衄的方法在后世医家和百姓中广为流传。

　　在古代，中医治疗鼻衄的方法多种多样，与现代医学有所不同。如果对中医感兴趣，想更深地了解中医的神秘之处，欢迎加入中医的学习之旅。在这个旅程中，可以发现中医治疗鼻出血的丰富经验和卓越成就，并了解中医学派的独特视角和哲学理念。这不仅可以拓宽医学知识和视野，也为维护身体健康和生活品质注入新的力量和智慧。当然，如果小朋友们在平时出现鼻出血时，一定要寻求大人或者医生的帮助，自己不要盲目进行治疗。

Wang Zhizhong Treats Nasal Bleeding with Moxibustion

Nose bleeding is a common experience for people. It can be caused by external injury or other factors, which may reflect the condition of the body to certain extent. Nose bleeding should be treated in time by pinching the nose with hands to coagulate the blood and keeping the head as forward as possible at the same time to avoid swallowing the blood which may irritate the gastrointestinal tract. If nose bleeding lasts for a long time or occurs frequently, it is recommended to seek medical treatment promptly. The doctor can find out the cause of the bleeding through meticulous examination and then formulate a treatment plan accordingly. The Chinese name for nose bleeding is "Bí Nǜ (epistaxis)". So how did people treat nose bleeding in ancient times? Here is the story about Wang Zhizhong, a famous ancient doctor, who treated nose bleeding with moxibustion.

Wang Zhizhong styled himself Shu Quan, was a famous acupuncturist and doctor in the Southern Song Dynasty. One day, his mother suffered from nose bleeding suddenly. As a doctor, Wang Zhizhong rushed to fill prescription and treat his mother with medicine based on his experience. To his surprise, the formula, which was effective for other patients, was of no avail for his mother's nose bleeding. Wang Zhizhong was very anxious and hurriedly looked through medical books to search for other treatments for this disease, hoping to relieve his mother's pain as soon as possible. After browsing through many books, he found such a sentence in the *Collection of Effective Prescriptions*, "The disease of bleeding from the mouth and nose is called cerebral epistaxis, which can be treated by applying 50 columns of moxa cone on the Shangxing acupoint (GV 23)". At first, Wang Zhizhong doubted the credibility of the book for its statement of applying 50 columns of moxa cone, because most of the acupoints on head could not be selected for moxibustion. But at this time there was no other better treatment method, so he had to treat his mother according to the book. To ensure safety, Wang Zhizhong burned 7 columns cautiously at first. The moxibustion was very effective for his mother's nose bleeding was stopped. Wang Zhizhong was very happy and deeply appreciated the greatness of Chinese medicine, keeping this method in mind. However, his mother's nose bleeding recurred the next day, Wang Zhizhong burned 14 columns on the acupoints of the head and the disease was cured without recurrence. From this case, Wang Zhizhong learned a good method for treating nose bleeding. Later, whenever he saw people suffering from nose bleeding, Wang Zhizhong would tell them the treatment method, namely, burning moxa cone on the Xinhui and Shangxing acupoint of the head, and then the disease would be relieved till cured. This method of treating nose bleeding was widely spread among people and doctors in later generations.

There are various methods to treat nose bleeding in Chinese medicine, which are quite different from modern medicine. If you are interested in Chinese medicine and want to learn more about the mysteries of it, you are welcome to join the journey of learning Chinese medicine. In this journey, you can find out the rich experience and remarkable achievements of TCM in treating nose bleeding and learn about the unique perspective and philosophy of the TCM. This will not only broaden our medical knowledge and vision, but also inject new strength and wisdom to our health cultivation and life quality. Of course, if you have nose bleeding in daily life, seek help from adults or doctors instead of treating it blindly.

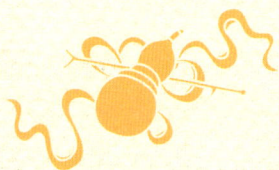

笔针治愈公主喉痈

　　在古代，有一位公主生病了，她的喉咙里长了一个很大的脓包，每日疼痛难忍，吃不下饭。皇帝看着她的宝贝女儿日渐消瘦的身体和被病痛折磨的样子心里很难受，命人召来皇宫里最好的医生给公主治病。医生说公主的病需要用针刀划开脓包，里面的脓液才会流出来，疾病才会痊愈。奈何公主闻此便惊恐大哭，不愿进行治疗。看着脓包一天天地变大，再这样下去，公主可能会被饿死啊。皇帝对此心急如焚，不知如何是好。正当皇帝焦急万分的时候，身边的

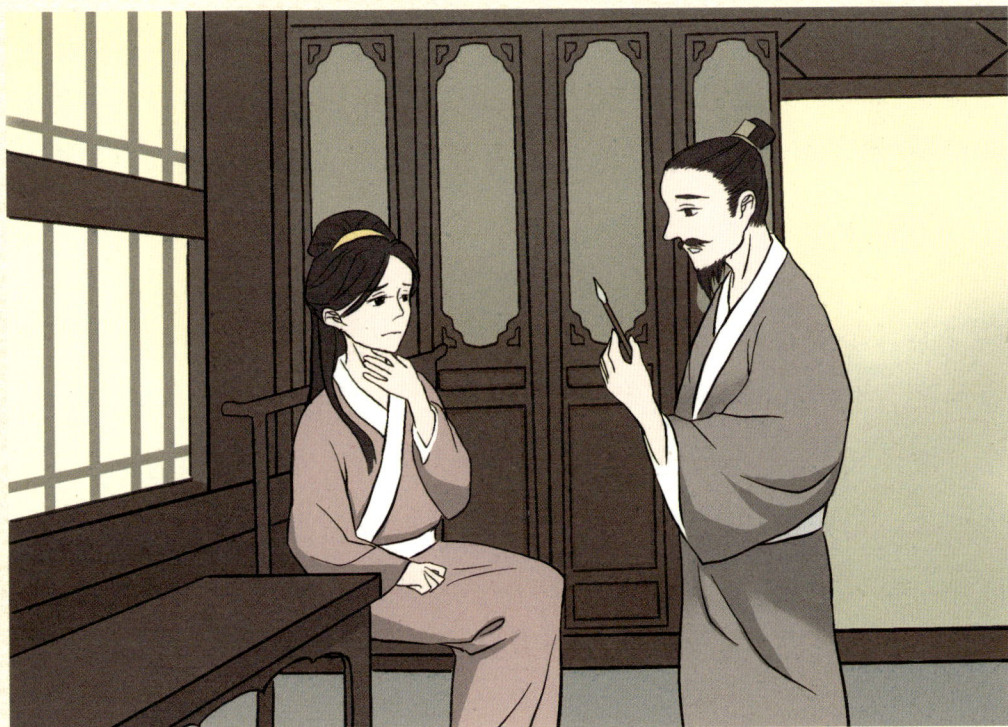

大臣给出了一个主意，让皇帝下旨，从民间寻找医生来治疗公主的疾病。没过几天，一位卖药的民间医生来到皇宫，说："我不用针刀便可治好公主的疾病，只需要在药笔上蘸点药粉，然后涂抹在脓包上，脓包就会破溃。"公主一听不用针刀，高高兴兴地接受了这位医生的治疗。只见这位医生从随身携带的药箱中拿出一支药笔，一盒药粉，用药笔蘸取药粉后在公主喉咙的脓包上轻轻划了一下，脓包瞬间破溃，流出的脓液差不多有一茶杯那么多。公主瞬间自觉喉咙疼痛减轻，也可按时进食。

过了几天，公主喉咙上的脓包消失了，疾病也痊愈了。皇帝见此非常高兴，不仅要拿出重金来感谢这位医生，还要为他加官进爵。皇帝希望他能把治好公主的药方贡献出来，这位医生一听，连忙下跪，并说道："希望皇帝不要怪罪于我，我用的药粉其实就是普通的药粉，也不是什么秘方，因为听说公主害怕针刀，所以我就在我的药笔中藏了一根很细的针，当我用药笔将药粉涂在脓包上的那一刻，针也会瞬间划破脓包，这样一来，公主不用害怕，同时也成功地进行了治疗。"皇帝听后恍然大悟，大赞其医术之高明。最终这位医生向皇帝请辞，又开始了他走街串巷，治病救人的走方医生活。

在人们交流的过程中，真诚确实是必不可少的，但还是需要一些"谎言"的存在，它有时候可以作为人际关系的润滑剂，是"善意的谎言"。故事中的医生就说了一个"善意的谎言"，如果不是这个"谎言"，公主有可能会一直拒绝接受治疗，最终会因为吃不下饭而死去，皇帝则会因为失去心爱的女儿而痛苦万分，医生"善意的谎言"避免了这一切的发生。所以，只要在人际交往的过程中分清场合，掌握时机，那么"善意的谎言"是可以存在的。

The Treatment of Throat Abscess for the Princess with Needle in Brush Pen

In ancient times, there was a princess who was seriously ill near death with abscess in her throat, making her unable to take any food. The emperor sent for the imperial physician to treat the princess, who said that the disease needs to be treated by cutting the throat abscess open to let out the pus and blood firstly, and then applying medicine on the wound. When the princess heard this, she cried in horror and refused to be treated. The throat abscess was getting worsened day by day, and if it continues like this, the princess might starve to death. The emperor was anxious and had no idea about how to deal with it. At this time, the ministers around the emperor suggested him to post a notice to find doctors from the common people to treat the princess's illness. A few days later, a folk doctor who lived by selling medication came to the palace and said, "I can cure the princess' disease without acupotomy. I just need to dip some medicinal powder with the brush pen and apply it on the throat abscess. The pus and blood will be removed." When the princess heard that there was no need for needles and knives, she happily accepted the doctor's treatment. The doctor took out a brush pen, dipped some medicinal powder from the box he carried, and gently scratched it on the throat abscess of the princess. The throat abscess burst instantly, the pus and blood flowed out almost as much as a teacup. The princess instantly felt relief in her throat, and she could eat as usual.

After a few days, the throat abscess of the princess disappeared and the disease was cured. The emperor was very happy and took out a lot of money to thank the doctor, and gave the official position and knight title to the doctor with the hope that he could contribute the method and formula to the imperial hospital. When the doctor heard this, he quickly knelt down and said, "Please forgive me. The medicinal powder used is actually ordinary instead of a secret recipe. I heard that the princess is afraid to be treated by needle knives, so I hid a very thin needle in the brush pen. When I applied the powder on the throat abscess with the brush pen, the needle cut through the pustules instantly. In this way, the princess was not frightened, and the disease was cured at the same time." After hearing this, the emperor understood the treatment thoroughly and praised his medical skills. In the end, the doctor resigned from the emperor and continued his work as a doctor who walked around the countryside to treat patients and save people.

In the process of interpersonal communication, sincerity is indeed essential. But sometimes certain lies are also necessary to be used as a lubricant for interpersonal relationships which are called "white lies". In the above story, the doctor told a white lie to save the life of the princess. Without this lie, the princess might have refused to receive treatment and eventually died of starvation. The emperor would be in great pain because of the loss of his beloved daughter. All these tragedies were prevented by the doctor's white lie. Therefore, white lies are significant when applied in proper occasion and moment during the process of interpersonal communication.

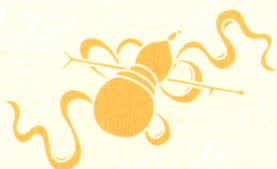

李东垣刺印堂出血治眩晕

　　在金元时期，有一位医家名叫李东垣，他自小便聪明好学，学习了我国的许多经典著作。就在他十八岁那一年，他的母亲突然生病了，李东垣每天都陪伴在母亲身边，照顾母亲，并且苦寻名医以求救治母亲。这个时期的医生们对疾病的见识广泛，各执己见，尽管请了很多医生给他的母亲开了很多药，但喝下后病情就是不见好转，最后很遗憾，他的母亲去世了。这件事情对李东垣的影响很大，自此他便走上了学医的道路。他成为了名医张元素的学生，由于他

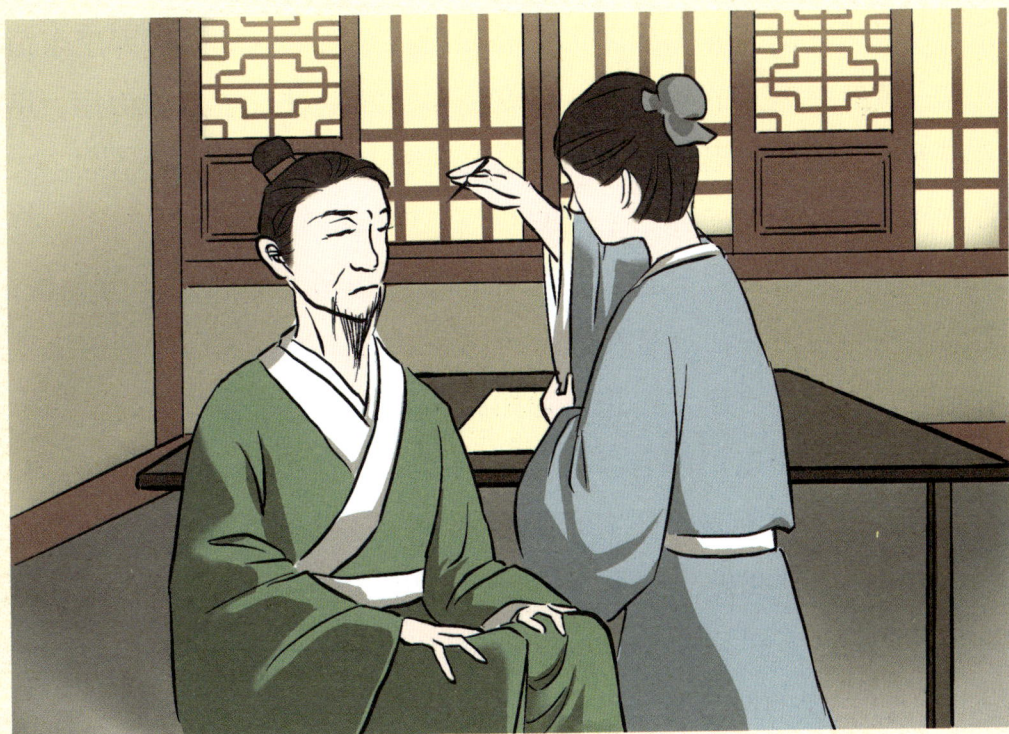

自小博览群书，又跟着名师在临床上认真学习，所以他很快便掌握了老师教给他的所有知识，并且李东垣在后来医学上取得的成就远超过他的老师，他将自己对疾病的认识和相关的治疗方法写成了书，好让后世进行学习。他的主要著作有《脾胃论》《内外伤辨惑论》等，均对中医学的发展产生了深远的影响。

有一年春天，一位老人来找李东垣看病，他已经快七十岁了，只见他面部很红，就好像喝了酒似的，他告诉李东垣说自己最近吐出来的痰很黏稠，并且有时候会感觉到头晕目眩，就好像在天上飞，穿梭在风云之间，视力也越来越差，有时候甚至看不到东西。李东垣听完老人的描述之后，就开始为老人把脉，通过把脉李东垣知晓了老人是很明显的上热下寒，他便想使用寒凉药，但是又考虑到老人现在的年龄，身体已经很虚弱了，不能轻易使用寒凉药，这可怎么办呢？李东垣想起老师跟他说过，治疗上焦的疾病，就好像是一群乌鸦聚集在高高的山巅之上，需要用箭来射取乌鸦。随即李东垣便拿三棱针在老人的额头部，也就是印堂穴上进行了点刺治疗，迅速刺了二十余次，出血大概四十毫升时，老人便觉得头目清利，之前的各种症状都消失了，后来再也没有复发过。

从这个病案可以看出，李东垣在诊治患者的过程中十分谨慎，不会随意使用药物，只有在综合考虑患者的体质状况后才会决定使用何种方法进行治疗，正是因为如此，老人的病才会痊愈。试想一下，如果当时李东垣没有考虑老人的体质而直接使用了寒凉药物，说不定疾病不但不减轻还有可能会加重。这就告诉人们一个道理，在生活中，当需要做出一个决定或者得出一个结论的时候，一定不能太过于武断，必须要经过深思熟虑。人们耳熟能详的一句话"三思而后行"，说的便是这个道理。

Li Dongyuan Treats Vertigo by Needling Yintang to Let Blood

Li Dongyuan, a physician in the Jin Yuan period, was smart and studious when he was a child, reading many classic works. When he was eighteen years old, his mother suddenly fell ill. So Li Dongyuan began to accompany his mother every day, taking care of her and searching for famous doctors to treat her disease. Doctors in this period had a wide range of knowledge and held their own opinions about the disease. Although Li Dongyuan asked many doctors to prescribe drugs for his mother, her condition was not improved. In the end, his mother passed away pitifully. Influenced by the doctors, Li Dongyuan started to learn medicine. He became a student of the famous doctor Zhang Yuansu. Because he had read many books since childhood and learned diligently from famous doctors in clinical practice. Li Dongyuan mastered all the knowledge taught to him by the teacher. His later achievements in medicine far exceeded those of his teacher. He documented his understanding of the disease and related treatment methods in the book for future generations to study. His main works include *Treatise on Spleen and Stomach*, *Clarifying Doubts about Damage from Internal and External Causes*, etc. These books have a far-reaching impact on the development of Chinese medicine.

One spring, an old man came to seek help from Li Dongyuan. He was almost seventy years old, and his face was very red as if he had drunk alcohol. The old man said that the phlegm he spit out was very sticky, and he felt dizzy sometimes just like flying in the sky and shuttling across wind and cloud. He said his eyesight was becoming worse and worse, even blind sometimes. After hearing his description, Li Dongyuan began to take his pulse and knew that he had a heat syndrome which should be treated with cold medicine in property. However, considering the old man's age and weak body, cold medicine in property could not be used easily. How to solve it? Li Dongyuan remembered that his teacher had told him treating the disease of upper energizer was like facing a flock of crows gathering on a high mountaintop. The method is to shoot the crows with arrows. Li Dongyuan took out a three-edged needle immediately to prick the old man's Yintang acupoint for more than 20 times to let about forty milliliters of blood. After that, the old man felt the eyesight was clear and the previous symptoms were gone. His disease never recurred later.

From this story we can see that Li Dongyuan was very cautious in the process of diagnosing and treating diseases. He did not use drugs at will. On the contrary, he would analyze the patient's physical condition comprehensively before deciding the method for treatment. Thanks for this, the old man's disease was cured eventually. If Li Dongyuan did not consider the old man's physique condition at that time and used cold medicine directly, the disease would not have been alleviated but aggravated. This tells us that we should not be arbitrary but be very cautious before making a decision or drawing a conclusion. There is truth in the saying: Think twice before acting.

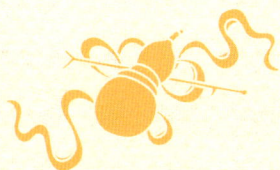

罗天益针灸治小儿痫证

　　元朝时期，有一户魏姓人家，家里有一个四岁大的小儿子，暂且叫他小魏。小魏生了一场很奇怪的病，但幸运的是遇到了一位医术精湛的医生，最后治好了这个奇怪的病。

　　这户人家素来信佛，他们希望小魏平安健康地长大。有一天，他们去寺庙请来一群僧人为小魏举办祈福活动。这些僧人全都身穿黑色衣服，聚在小魏身边，刚开始念咒，小魏就被吓得突然大哭，怎么哄他都没用，然后嘴巴里面开始吐出白色的痰液，眼睛也往上

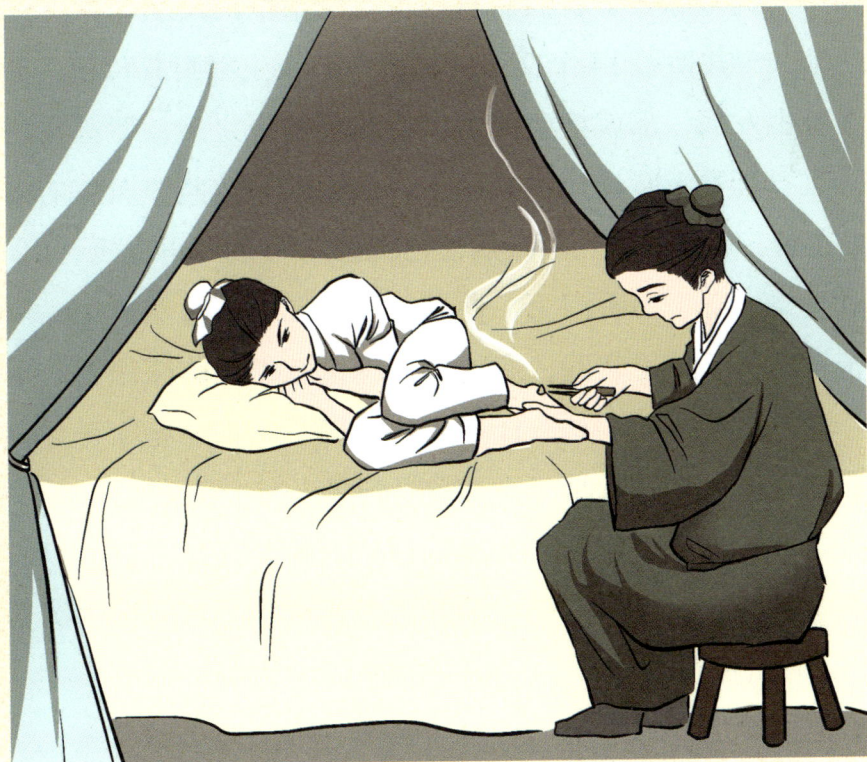

翻，身体蜷曲，喉咙里面还发出"吼吼"的响声，过了一阵才醒过神来。自此之后，小魏一看到穿黑色衣服的人，这个奇怪的病就开始发作。他的家人为此很是着急，也找了很多医生。这些医生们大都给他吃一些重镇安神的中药，比如朱砂、犀角、龙骨、牡蛎等。吃了这些药后，大概过了四十天左右，家里人发现小魏的病情非但没有好转，又出现了一些新的症状，他走路的姿势和思考的神态越来越像痴呆的样子。家人看在眼里，急在心上，赶紧遍寻名医，于是请到了一位非常优秀的医生——罗天益。

罗医生经过把脉，发现小魏的脉象很沉很急，并且像弹琴弦似的，立马想到自己读过的医书里面有对这些症状的相关描述。利用书里面的知识，罗医生很快知道了小魏得"怪病"的原因，并且很快给出了相应的治疗方案。罗医生吩咐随从制作了艾炷，把其中一个放在小魏的申脉穴上，然后点燃，艾灸部位的皮肤微微发红时就再换一个，一共换了 14 个艾炷。之后，罗医生嘱咐其母道，如果下次是在晚上发病，那就换灸照海穴。艾灸结束之后，罗医生对症下药，并煎煮沉香天麻汤让小魏服下。之后家人按照罗医生的嘱咐悉心照顾小魏，服用三副药后疾病便已痊愈，"怪病"再也没有出现过。

罗天益出身于书香门第，性情敦厚，自小便博览群书，对待医学刻苦钻研，且勤于实践，有扎实的理论知识和临床积累。尽管人们都夸赞其医术高超，他仍旧"恨所业未精"，时常抱有谦虚谨慎的治学态度，也正因为如此，罗天益得到了当时一位中医大家，"金元四大家"之一李杲的赏识，并得以拜他为师。在此之后，罗天益致力于对李杲医学著作的整理和学术思想的传播，对后世中医学的发展做出了巨大的贡献。

Luo Tianyi Treated Pediatric Epilepsy with Acupuncture

During the Yuan Dynasty, there was a family surnamed Wei with a four-year-old son, who was temporarily called Xiao Wei. Xiao Wei once suffered from a very strange disease and was luckily cured by a skilled doctor.

The family believed in Buddhism and hoped that Xiao Wei would grow up safely and healthily. One day, they invited a group of monks from the temple to hold a blessing. But Xiao Wei was frightened greatly and cried suddenly when these black-dressed monks gathered around him to chant the mantra. He cried and couldn't be comforted. Then, his mouth began to spit out white sputum, his eyes rolled upward, his body curled, and his throat gave out roaring sound. It took a while for him to wake up. Since then, Xiao Wei would suffer from the same symptoms as whenever he saw black-dressed people. His family were very anxious and invited many doctors to treat him. Most of these doctors prescribed medicinal herbs to calm his mind such as cinnabar, rhinoceros horn, fossil fragment and oyster, etc. After taking these medicines for about forty days, the family found that Xiao Wei's condition was not improved but worsened with some new symptoms. His posture and cognitive abilities increasingly resembled those of someone with dementia. The family were very worried and searched for famous doctors all around. Finally, they invited a very excellent doctor named Luo Tianyi for Xiao Wei.

After checking his pulse, Luo Tianyi found that Xiao Wei's pulse was very heavy and rapid like playing a string. Based on the description of syndromes recorded in the medical books, Luo immediately figured out the cause of Xiao Wei's "strange disease" and quickly decided the therapeutic schedule. Luo instructed his attendants to make several moxa cones and burn one of them on Xiao Wei's Shenmai acupoint. When the skin around the acupoint was slightly red, he replaced a new moxa cone to continue the moxibustion. It took 14 moxa cones for the treatment. After that, Luo told his mother that if the disease occurred again at night, she should use moxibustion on the Zhaohai acupoint. Additionally, Luo prescribed medicinal herbs and prepared Chenxiang Tianma Tang (Agilawood and GastrodiaTuber Decoction) for Xiao Wei to take. The family took good care of Xiao Wei according to Luo's instructions, and the disease was cured after taking three doses without recurrence.

Luo Tianyi was born in a scholarly family and read extensively since childhood. He was good-natured, hard-working in learning medical knowledge and diligent in medical practice. With solid theoretical knowledge and clinical accumulation, he was recognized as superb in medical skills. But he was very modest and cautious in academic pursuit, and held the attitude of "worrying about the imperfect proficiency" for continuous self-improvement. As a result, Luo Tianyi was appreciated by Li Gao, one of the "Four Great Physicians in Jin Yuan Dynasty", and had the opportunity to learn from him as a student. Afterwards, Luo Tianyi devoted himself to the collation and dissemination of Li Gao's medical works and academic ideas, and made great contributions to the development of Chinese medicine in later generations.

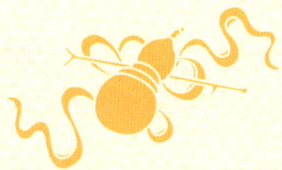

徐文中治疗镇南王妃卧床不起

　　元朝有位医家名叫徐文中，字用和，是宣州人。他从岳父那里继承了针灸、中药、方剂、术数，又擅长画符写咒，因此渐渐在江湖上有了名气。有一次他出门游历，到了吴郡这个地方，恰好遇到吴郡有个大户人家因沾染湿气而得了腿病，这户人家就请徐文中来治疗。徐文中为患者针刺治疗之后，病即刻就好了，于是徐文中被留在当地做郡吏。

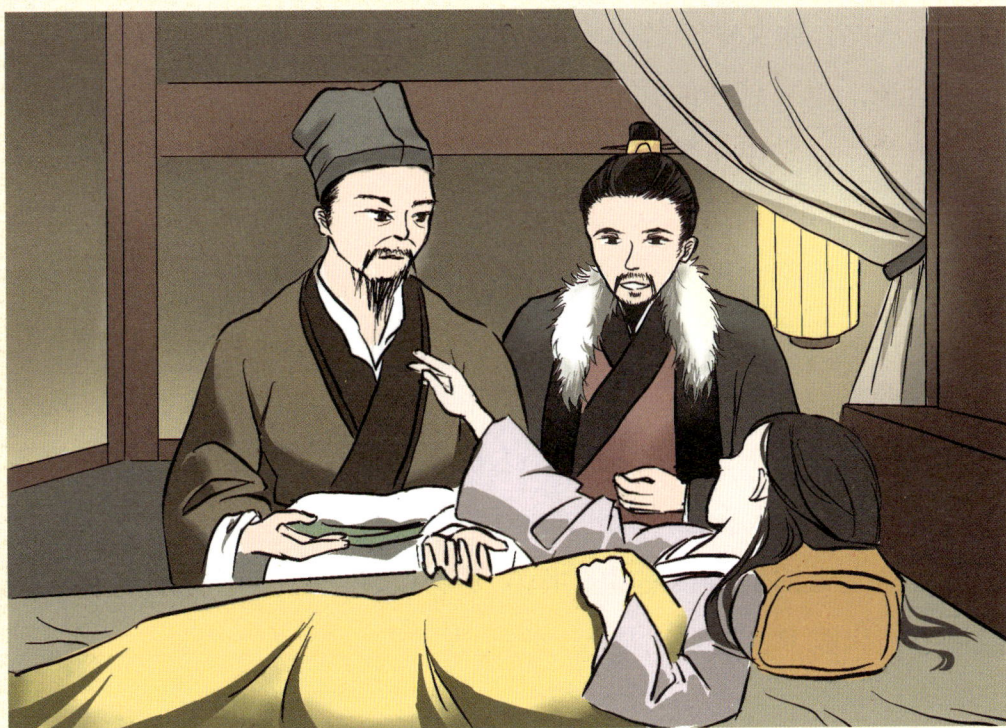

当时，镇南王的王妃卧病在床，病得很重，以至于没法从床上坐起来。王府里的御医费尽心思医治，但都没能治好王妃的病。南台有一名叫秃鲁的侍御史听说徐文中医术高明，就向镇南王推荐了他。镇南王听说后立即派人驾着马车飞奔去吴郡请徐文中。徐文中到后，镇南王以礼相待，赐他坐到偏殿谈话，跟他讲述了王妃的病情，并请他进入内室为王妃诊查。

徐文中请王妃抬起手足，王妃却说抬不起来，在仔细地诊查后，徐文中按压住王妃手上的合谷、曲池两穴，随即进针，针法高超，王妃一点痛的感觉都没有。针灸了一会，徐文中再次请王妃举起双手，王妃又推辞说抬不起来。徐文中解释道："手上的针气已经运行了。请您抬手试一试。"王妃试了一下，果然手能够举起来了，又请她抬脚，脚也能够抬起来了，镇南王见状异常欣喜。到了第二天，王妃能从床上坐起来了。镇南王大摆筵席，赏赐了徐文中数不清的钱财。从此，徐文中的名声响彻广陵，大家都以为他是扁鹊在世。

后来，越来越多的达官显贵听说徐文中医术高明，都来请他治病。因此，徐文中虽然官职不大，但家境日益富饶。他曾经对一位朋友说道："我门下弟子众多，然而没有一个弟子像我的医术一样出神入化，他们都贪图功名利禄而不知道礼义。我凭借着我这医术游历江湖，前前后后四十多年了，我所治好的患者不计其数，而我从来没有要求他们回报我，我只知道用我的医术治病救人罢了。现如今有幸得到了上天给我的福报，达官显贵赏赐给我的东西我推辞不掉，对于贫穷的人我也从来不敢不尽心治疗。"

从徐文中的话可以看出，医生要有仁爱之心，不贪图名利，才能潜心钻研医术，达到出神入化的境界。

Xu Wenzhong Treated the Bed-ridden Zhennan Princess

In the Yuan Dynasty, there was a doctor named Xu Wenzhong, also known as Yonghe, who was from Xuanzhou. He learned the skills of acupuncture and moxibustion, Chinese medicine, prescription, divination and incantation from his father-in-law, gaining increasing popularity in the society. Once he travelled for pleasure and got to Wujun, where he happened to cure the leg disease caused by dampness promptly for a patient from a wealthy family with acupuncture. So Xu Wenzhong was asked to stay in the local region as a magistrate.

At that time, the princess of the King of Zhennan was seriously ill, unable to sit up from bed. The imperial physicians in the palace of the prince tried their best to treat the princess but in vain. An official from Nantai Province named Tu Lu heard about Xu Wenzhong's superb medical skills and recommended him to the King of Zhenan, who sent for Xu Wenzhong immediately from Wujun. When Xu Wenzhong arrived, the King of Zhenan treated him with due respect and talked with him in the side hall, telling him about the princess's illness and inviting him inside to diagnose disease for the princess.

Xu Wenzhong asked the princess to lift her hands and feet, but the princess said that she could not lift them. After careful examination, Xu Wenzhong pressed the Hegu and Quchi acupoint of the princess' hand, and inserted the needle skillfully without producing any pain. After treating her with acupuncture for a while, Xu Wenzhong again asked the princess to lift her hands, but the princess said the same words again. Xu Wenzhong explained, "The qi of your hands is already circulating normally, please have a try to lift your hands." The princess tried and really raised her hands and feet successfully. The King of Zhennan was very delighted. By the next day, the princess had been able to sit up from bed. The King of Zhennan gave a big feast and rewarded Xu Wenzhong with countless amounts of money. Since then, Xu Wenzhong became well-known in Guangling and was regarded as Bianque reborn.

Later, more and more important officials and wealthy people heard about Xu Wenzhong's excellent medical skills and invited him to treat their diseases. Therefore, Xu Wenzhong's family became increasingly rich though his official position was not very high. He once said to a friend, "I have a large number of disciples, but none of them is as superb as me in medical skills. They are all in pursuit of fame and fortune, but have no idea about the propriety and righteousness. I have traveled around the world and treated numerous patients with my medical skills for more than 40 years. I never asked them to return the favor, just treating diseases with my medical skills. Now I am blessed with all these favors. I can not turn down the rewards from high-ranking officials and wealthy people, but I always dedicate myself in treating diseases for the poor."

From Xu Wenzhong's words, we can learn that only with a heart of benevolence and a strong will to keep away from fame and fortune, can the doctors devote themselves to the study of medical skills and reach the acme of perfection.

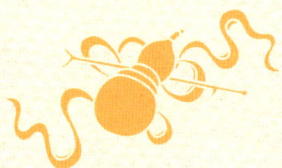

凌云针刺治疗咳嗽

　　《明史》中记载了一位颇负盛名的针灸医家，名叫凌云，字汉章，是浙江归安人。他曾经是一名生员，后来放弃学业，向北而去，游历泰山。相传有位道士在一座古庙里传授给凌云一套神奇的针灸医术，治疗疾病没有不见效的。

　　有一天，凌云听说有个同乡人咳嗽的非常严重，已经有整整五天的时间吃不下东西了，他的家人为他请了多名大夫诊治，病情不但没好转反而越来越严重。凌云心想："这位患者恐怕快撑不住了，我赶紧去看看，或许能有所帮助。"

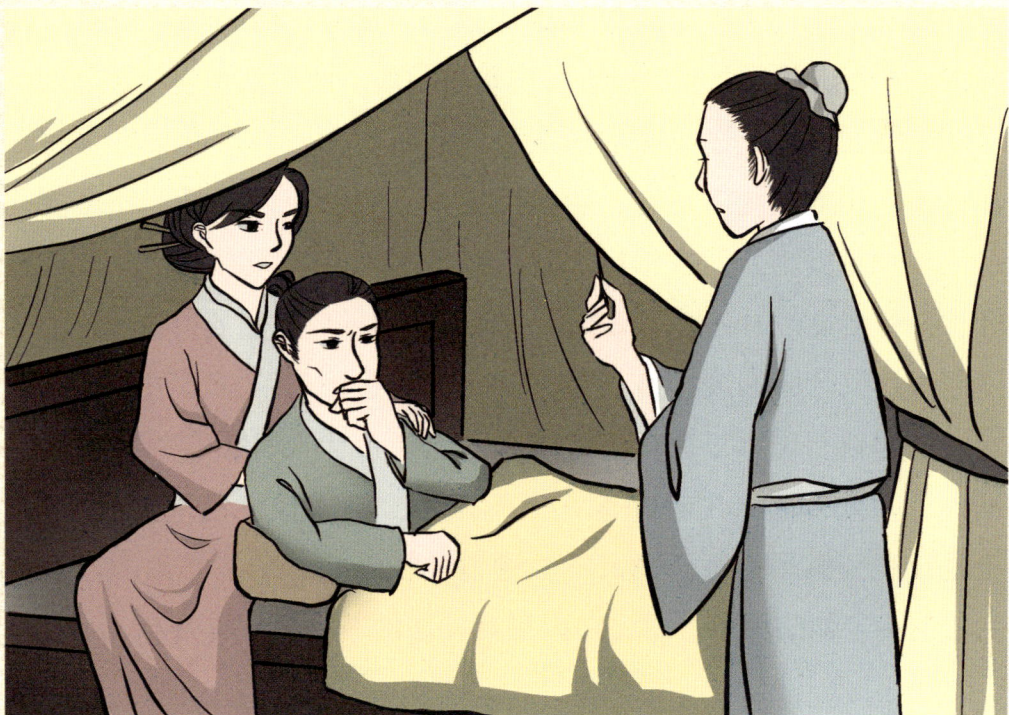

凌云仔细诊察患者的病情，心中已有判断，再细细察看其他大夫诊治后开的药方，发现一个规律，每个大夫开的药方虽然有所差异，但是都是补益的药物，患者服下之后，病情反而更重了。凌云把自己的看法讲给患者家属听，并进一步解释道："通过诊察病情，我发现他的病是寒湿郁积所导致的，之前的大夫没有看到他病情的真正病因，所以开的药方无法治疗他的病证。"

家属问凌云："那您能治好他的病吗？"凌云说："我可以用针灸的方法治好他的病，不过，要施针的穴位在他的头顶，依照他现在的情况，头部施针的刺激会比较大，他可能会因为刺激太大而晕过去，但你们不用担心，他一会儿就能醒过来。在我治疗的时候需要四个人往不同方向拉住他的头发，以固定住头部，防止倾斜。"

患者的头部固定好后，凌云开始全神贯注地施针，之后患者果然晕厥过去，家属们担心地哭泣。凌云颇为自信，让患者家属不用担心。过了一会了，患者果然苏醒过来。这时，凌云再次施针，行补法，接着出针。之后，患者咳出很多的痰，咳嗽就慢慢痊愈了。

从凌云治疗上述咳嗽的医案可以看出，任何治疗方案都要建立在诊断正确的前提下进行，否则，不仅不利于疾病康复，还可能耽误或者加重病情。而在治疗的过程中，离不开胆大心细，既要对施针过程和结果心中有数，又要关注到患者的反应及家属的感受。

孝宗皇帝听闻凌云有一手绝妙针法，在民间治好了很多疑难杂症，就把他召进宫里来，下旨考验他。皇帝让太医把衣服穿在针灸铜人上，要求凌云用针在铜人上刺出考到的穴位，结果全部正确，于是让凌云做了御医。凌云不断通过他精湛的针法治病救人，他的后代继承了他的医术，四海之内提到针法的，大家都称赞归安凌氏。

Ling Yun Treats Cough with Acupuncture

It is recorded in the *History of Ming Dynasty* that there was a famous acupuncturist named Ling Yun, with the style name of Hanzhang and from Gui'an, Zhejiang Province. He was once a scholar, but gave up his studies later and headed north to visit Mount Tai. According to legend, a Taoist priest taught Ling Yun a set of magical acupuncture skills in an ancient temple, which was very effective for treating diseases.

One day, Ling Yun heard that a fellow countryman suffered from a bad cough and had been unable to take food for five days. His family invited several doctors to treat him but in vain. Ling Yun thought that the patient was very dangerous and hurried to offer help.

Ling Yun examined the patient carefully and had his own judgement. He studied the medicines prescribed by other doctors and found that, though a little different, they were all herbs with tonifying function. The patient became worsened after taking the decoctions. Ling Yun explained his opinion to the patient's family and said, "After examining his disease, I found it was caused by accumulation of dampness and coldness. The previous doctors did not find out the real cause of his disease, so their prescriptions could not treat his syndrome."

The family member asked Ling Yun, "Can you cure his disease?"

Ling Yun said, "I can treat him with acupuncture on his head. He might lose consciousness because of the great stimulation from the needling therapy. But do not worry, he will wake up soon. During the acupuncture, I need four persons to hold his hair in four directions to keep his head fixed to avoid tilting. "

After the patient's head was put still, Ling Yun began to concentrate on the acupuncture treatment. Then, the patient fainted as expected and the family were worried to cry. Ling Yun was quite confident, talking and laughing freely, and let the family relaxed. After a while, the patient really woke up. At this time, Ling Yun inserted the needles again with tonifying method, and then withdrew the needles. After that, the patient kept vomiting much phlegm, and his cough was gradually cured.

From the above medical case, it can be seen that any treatment plan should be based on correct diagnosis, otherwise it will delay and even aggravate the disease, let alone cure the disease. And in the process of treatment, the doctor needs to be bold but cautious, having confidence in the treatment and effect of acupuncture, and showing concern for the patient's response and the family's feeling.

When Emperor XiaoZong of Ming Dynasty heard about the magical acupuncture skill of Ling Yun that had cured many difficult miscellaneous diseases in folk, he summoned him to the palace to test him. The emperor let the imperial physician put clothes on the acupuncture bronze figure and asked Ling Yun to needle the named acupoints of the figure examined. Ling Yun needled accurately and was appointed as an imperial physician. Ling Yun treated and saved a lot of people continuously with his superb needling skill. His medical skills were inherited by his later descendants. It was praised that Master Ling of Gui'an by everyone when acupuncture was discussed around the nation.

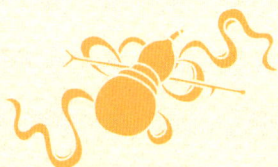

医学巨著《针灸大成》问世

　　《针灸大成》是明朝时期的一本针灸学专著，这本书面世 400 多年来，到目前已有 70 多个版本，被翻译成日、法、德等多种语言，它对针灸学术在中国乃至全世界的传播都起到了积极的推动作用，至今仍被奉为针灸学习者的必备之书。它的出版有着一段曲折动人的故事。

　　这本书的原作者是明代著名针灸医家杨继洲，他在经过长期实践积累了丰富的治疗经验的基础上，将祖传秘方与自己的经验结合

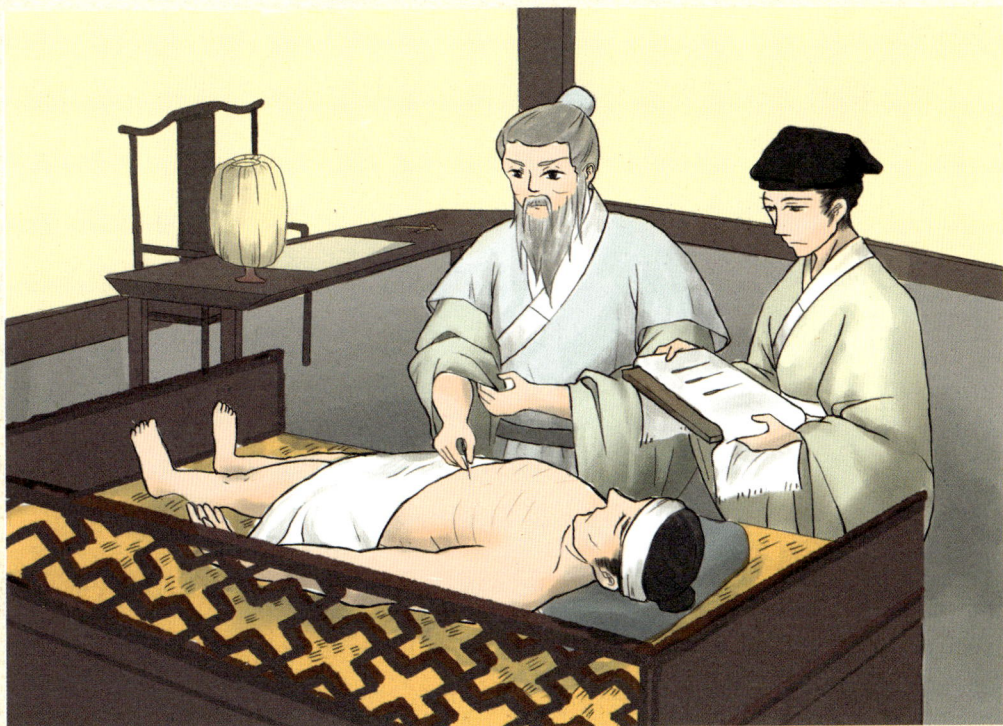

起来，编成了一本书——《卫生针灸玄机秘要》，还请了当时吏部尚书王国光为这本书做了序言。他希望这本书能出版发行，让针灸医术得到传播，以便为更多的人解除病痛，可惜他的愿望一直没能实现。

正当杨继洲为此事烦恼的时候，他碰到了一位极为特殊的患者。那是明万历年间，有位巡按山西监察御史叫赵文炳，他不幸患上"痿痹之疾"，突发身体一侧瘫痪，胳膊、腿儿都不能动了，遍请名医，吃了无数的药，可惜均无任何疗效。正在这位高官心急如焚，一筹莫展之际，有人推荐了一位精通针灸医术并且名满京城的太医——杨继洲，他曾为多位王公大臣治好过疑难重病，其祖父也是太医。杨继洲从北京一路赶来山西，经过一番望闻问切，为赵文炳扎下三根银针。仅仅用了三根针，瘫痪卧床的赵文炳竟奇迹般地站了起来，先前的症状也都消失殆尽。这使饱受疾病困扰的赵文炳如释重负，喜不自胜。

赵文炳看了杨继洲随身携带的医书《卫生针灸玄机秘要》，深刻体会到针灸是疗效神奇的医术，值得大力推广。此外，当时杨继洲已是近八十岁的老人，一路翻山越岭，长途跋涉，不辞辛苦地专程从北京赶来为赵文炳治病，这份深情厚意，让赵文炳对他感激涕零。为了答谢杨继洲，决定帮他付印《卫生针灸玄机秘要》。眼看多年的愿望马上就可以实现，此时的杨继洲反倒不着急了。他静下心来，结合自己多年经验，重新审视历代各种针灸书籍。他要趁这次机会，好好地整理出一本有价值的针灸书籍出来。最后，他以自己的《卫生针灸玄机秘要》为基础，采集收录各地有关针灸的医书。同时请来能工巧匠雕刻针灸铜人雕像，刻板画图，详细标记经脉穴位。经过此番内容的扩大充实，最终编成了十卷二十余万字的《针灸大成》。

公元 1601 年，该书正式刊行。杨继洲三针治愈痿痹之疾的传奇故事也被赵文炳本人记录在为《针灸大成》一书所作的序言中，成为后世研究《针灸大成》成书的主要原始资料，也成为医患关系的美谈。

　　试想一下，如果没有杨继洲妙手仁心，三根银针治好赵文炳的怪病，也就可能不会有《针灸大成》这部针灸巨著；如果没有赵文炳对杨继洲知恩图报，资助杨继洲出版学术著作，也不会有《针灸大成》的问世。一位妙手仁心的医生，一位知恩图报的患者，这是医患关系的一段佳话，伴随着《针灸大成》的传播而深入人心。

The Story of the Medical Masterpiece
Compendium of Acupuncture and Moxibustion

Compendium of Acupuncture and Moxibustion is a specialized classic book on acupuncture and moxibustion published 400 years ago in the Ming Dynasty. It has more than 70 editions and has been translated into Japanese, French, German and many other languages. This classic book has made great contributions to the spread of acupuncture and moxibustion in China and around the world. It is still regarded as the indispensable authority to people who want to learn acupuncture and moxibustion up to now. Now, let's read a moving story about its publication.

The author of this book is Yang Jizhou, a famous physician in the Ming Dynasty. His dream was to combine traditional remedy with his own experience based on his long-term medical practice. Hence, he compiled a book named *Arcane Essentials of the Acupuncture and Moxibustion to Protect Health* and invited Wang Guoguang, a senior official of the Ministry, of personnel, to write a preface for this book. He hoped that the book could be published and read by more people, so their diseases could be treated and cured by acupuncture and moxibustion. However, his book was not published for some reason, and his dream was not realized. What a pity!

At this time, Yang Jizhou met a special patient named Zhao Wenbing. He was a supervisory censor of Shanxi province during the Wanli period of the Ming Dynasty. Zhao Wenbing suffered a lot from flaccidity paralysis and could not move his body and limbs freely. He had consulted many famous doctors and taken countless drugs, but his disease was not cured yet, which made this high-ranking official very worried. Then, Yang Jizhou was recommended to him as a well-known imperial physician skilled in acupuncture and moxibustion. It was said that he cured many severe diseases of imperial princes and court ministers. Additionally, it was said that the grandfather of Yang Jizhou was also an imperial physician. Therefore, Zhao Wenbing invited Yang Jizhou to treat his disease from Beijing to Shanxi. Yang Jizhou diagnosed his disease with the four methods firstly (namely, inspection, listening and smelling, inquiry, pulse-taking and palpation), and then gave him an acupuncture treatment by inserting three silver needles into his body. How amazing! The three silver needles took effect immediately, and Zhao Wenbing, once paralyzed and bedridden, could stand up miraculously! All his previous symptoms disappeared! This made Zhao Wenbing, who was troubled a lot by the disease, relieved and overjoyed.

After reading *Arcane Essentials of the Acupuncture and Moxibustion to Protect Health*, Zhao Wenbing realized that acupuncture was very effective in treating diseases, and it deserved large-scale promotion and spread. In addition, Yang Jizhou, as an eighty-year-old physician, came all the way from Beijing to Shanxi to help treat his disease despite the long distance and hardship of the journey. Zhao Wenbing was very grateful for the extreme kindness of Yang Jizhou, so he decided to help print the book written by Yang Jizhou. Knowing his dream would come true, Yang Jizhou was relieved and determined to re-examine various medical books on acupuncture and moxibustion in history and take this opportunity to compile a valuable book in this field. He collected and recorded relevant books from around the nation, and invited skillful craftsmen to sculp the bronze acupuncture status, cut blocks for printing, draw pictures and mark meridian acupoints on them in detail. Based on these preparations and his previous writings, the compilation of *Compendium of Acupuncture and Moxibustion* was completed successfully, consisting of ten volumes and more than 200000 words. In 1601, this great book was officially published and issued. This legendary story of treating flaccidity disease with three needles by Yang Jizhou was also recorded by Zhao Wenbing himself in the preface to the book. It has become the main source material for later generations to study this book, and a much-told story about the doctor-patient relationship.

Just imagine, *Compendium of Acupuncture and Moxibustion* would not be compiled if it weren't for Yang Jizhou's healing hands to cure Zhao Wenbing's disease with three needles, and it would not be published if it were not for Zhao Wenbing's financial support to show his deep gratitude to Yang Jizhou. The story between Yang Jizhou, a doctor with healing hands, and Zhao Wenbing, a grateful patient, is a good case in point to illustrate the doctor-patient relationship, and it has been deeply rooted in the hearts of the people with the spread of *Compendium of Acupuncture and Moxibustion.*

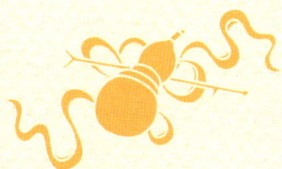

杨继洲针灸并用治好脾胃病

　　本篇故事出自明代的一部针灸学巨著——《针灸大成》，作者是杨继洲。他出身于中医世家，祖父是明朝的太医，家中有秘藏的医书秘籍，因为杨继洲对医学十分感兴趣，便拿出医书认真研读，最终精通针灸，其医术之高明广为流传。在杨继洲老年时期，他便决定写书论著，在家传医书的基础上，博览群书并结合自己的理论及经验，著成了《针灸大成》这本书，为后世针灸学发展做出了巨大的贡献。

　　有一天，杨继洲正在家中收拾院子里晒的草药，他的小徒弟从

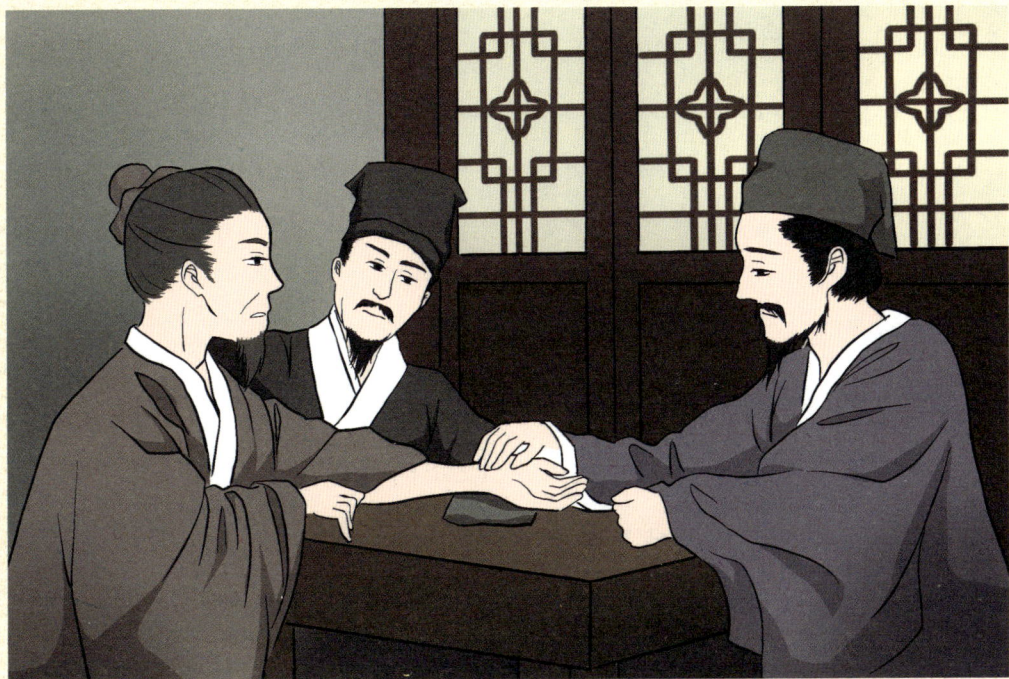

大门外跑进来，说是一位官员来访，想请杨继洲去为他的父亲诊病。官员见了杨继洲，向他说明了情况。原来官员父亲的肚子一直不舒服，还吃不下饭，这种症状已经持续了好长时间了。看着父亲难受的样子，官员心中很是担心，便一直照顾在父亲身边，在此期间广寻名医，尝试各种治疗方法，但是病情依旧未见好转。杨继洲感慨他的一片孝心，见官员一脸愁容，便立即和官员一同出发前去为其父亲诊病。杨继洲见到患者后，通过诊脉和倾听患者对症状的具体描述后，便诊断出患者是因为脾胃虚弱而导致肚子不舒服、吃不下饭等一系列症状。官员疑惑地看着杨继洲，问道："脾胃虚弱听着好像不是什么难治的病，但为什么我的父亲吃了好多药都不见好呢？"杨继洲耐心地解释道："如果把一个人想象成一棵大树，那么脾胃就是这棵大树的根基，所以脾胃对人来讲是很重要的，如果脾胃一旦出现问题，那就会有好多疾病随之出现，也正是因为它的重要性，所以对它的治疗也不是很简单啊。"听了杨继洲的解答，官员点了点头。随即，杨继洲对官员父亲进行了针刺加灸法的治疗，先用小艾炷灸穴位，然后再换用针刺，等灸的部位出现水疱，疾病也就慢慢恢复了。没过多久，杨继洲便收到官员的来信，说他的父亲疾病已经痊愈，现在身体恢复得非常好，信中还表达了对杨继洲的感谢和对其医术的钦佩。

　　通过这则故事可以了解到脾胃对身体健康的重要性，脾胃功能正常就可以将吃进去的食物转化为营养物质，从而让体质变得更强，这样就不容易生病了。那么应该如何保护脾胃呢？在日常生活中，要按时吃饭，按时睡觉，减少吃垃圾食品的次数，并且不能把肚子露在外面。通过平时养成的小习惯来保护好脾胃，保护好人体的根基。

Yang Jizhou Treats Spleen and Stomach Diseases with Acupuncture and Moxibustion

This story comes from *Compendium of Acupuncture and Moxibustion*, an acupuncture masterpiece written by Yang Jizhou in the Ming Dynasty. Yang Jizhou was born in a family of traditional Chinese medicine. His grandfather was an imperial doctor in the Ming Dynasty, so there were many medical books stored in the house. Yang Jizhou was very interested in medicine from childhood and did a lot of reading and study of medicine diligently. Finally, he became very proficient in acupuncture and was well-known for his superb medical skills. In his senior age, Yang Jizhou decided to write a treatise based on the medical books stored and his own theory and medical experience. Thus the book *Compendium of Acupuncture and Moxibustion* came out, which made great contributions to the development of acupuncture and moxibustion in later generations.

One day, Yang Jizhou was cleaning up the herbs dried in the yard when his little apprentice ran in and said that an official wanted to ask Yang Jizhou to diagnose his father. The official explained that his father has suffered disease related to stomach for a long time, which made his father unable to take any food. Being worried, the official took care of his father wholeheartedly and sent for many famous doctors but in vain. Yang Jizhou was moved by his filial piety and went with the official to diagnose his father immediately. After seeing the patient and diagnosing with pulse-taking and inquiry, Yang Jizhou concluded that it was the deficiency of spleen and stomach that caused the symptoms of the patient. Being doubtful, the official asked, "The deficiency of spleen and stomach sounds not difficult to treat. Why was my father not cured after taking a lot of medicine?" Yang Jizhou explained patiently, "If a person can be seen as a big tree, then the spleen and stomach are the foundation of this big tree, which are very important to us. If something is wrong with the spleen and stomach, diseases will occur. Therefore, it is not easy to treat diseases related with the spleen and stomach. " The official nodded. After the explanation, Yang Jizhou immediately treated the official's father with acupuncture and moxibustion. He heated the diseased part with moxa cone firstly, and then needled the acupoints involved. The patient felt better with blisters appearing at the diseased part. It didn't take long before Yang Jizhou received a letter from the official, saying that his father had recovered from his illness very well and expressing his gratitude and admiration to Yang Jizhou for his medical skills.

Through this story, we can understand the importance of the spleen and stomach to the health of the body. They can transform the food we eat into nutrients if they function normally. Then the physique will become stronger, and diseases will not occur easily. So how to protect our spleen and stomach? In daily life, we need to eat and sleep on time, reduce the taking of junk food, and keep the abdomen warm instead of being exposed. We should form good habits in daily life to protect our spleen and stomach function, which is the foundation of our body health.

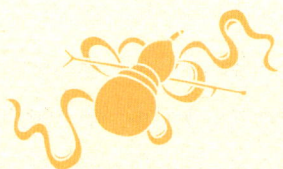

韩贻丰针刺治好中风

　　韩贻丰生活在清朝时期，是当时的一位县令，因为精通医术，便常常利用工作之余给人们诊病治病，医术之高明被广为流传。有一天，当地一位名叫徐元正的官员颜面部突然浮肿，嘴角一直流涎，说话含糊不清，就好像有东西堵在喉咙出不来，两条腿自觉像是绑了千斤重的石头抬不起来，连家里很低的门槛都难以跨过去。家人

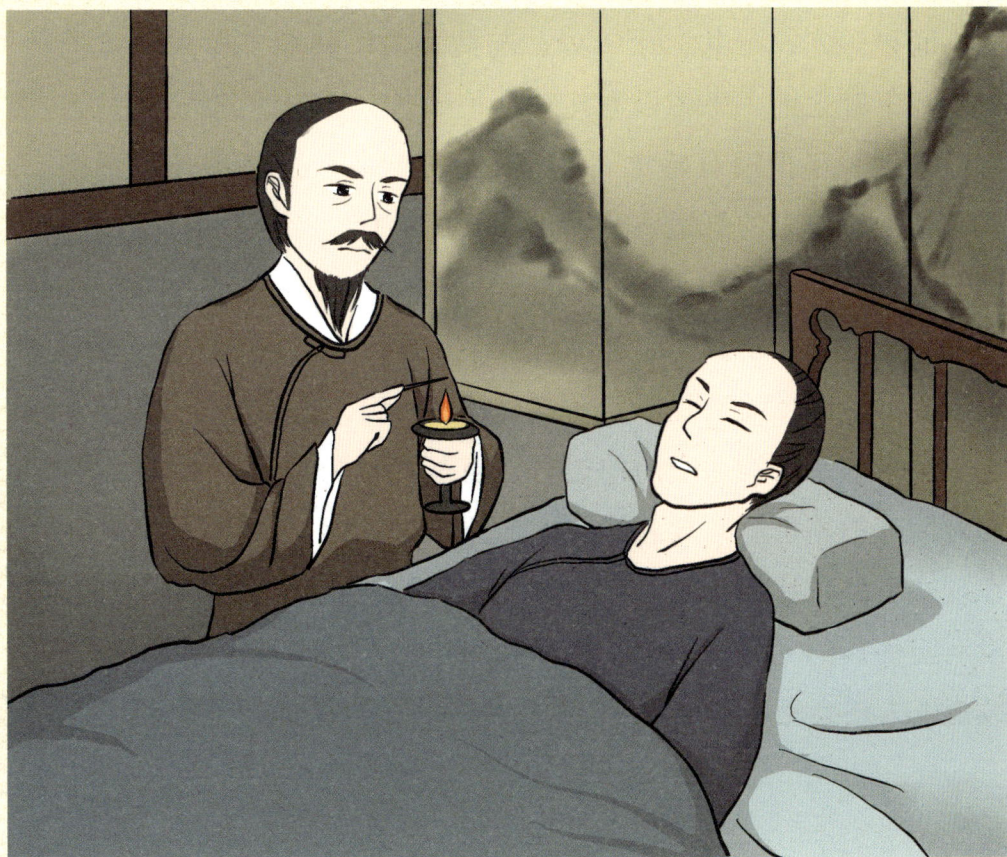

见此情形，便立马命人去请来韩贻丰为官员诊病。诊脉后，韩贻丰对其家人说："这个病必须要进行针刺才能治疗。"随即叫随从拿来烛台，放在患者头顶，拿出银针烧红准备针刺。官员及其孙子看到韩贻丰的此番操作都被吓得大惊失色，连连拒绝并说道："这里怎么能用火针呢，太危险了吧，这可使不得。"韩贻丰见此便给患者和家属解释这种治疗方法是安全的。无奈的是，几番解释下来，他们仍旧拒绝治疗，韩贻丰便离开了。几日后，徐元正的病愈发严重。这天，邻居前来看望徐元正，便建议道："听说县令韩贻丰的针灸技术非常了得，几乎全县的人都找他治病，你们可以请他来为大人看一看。"家人听罢，便再次邀请韩贻丰来诊病。韩贻丰不计前嫌，认真诊病，仍旧用火针针刺百会、神庭、肾俞、命门、环跳、风市、三里、涌泉等穴，一共二十一处。与此同时，韩贻丰命人煎煮汤药。在没有下针之前，患者以为扎针会很痛苦，等到针刺结束之后，患者惊喜地说不但没有感觉到疼痛，还在一阵阵煎药的药香熏陶下，有一种说不出来的舒适感。经过此次的治疗，徐元正的症状连同以前的小病一并消失了。

通过这个小故事，希望大家能够懂得，在人与人的交流过程中，要学会构建起"信任"这一道桥梁。医生诊病，患者看病，归根结底，也是医生和患者沟通交流的过程，有些患者因为对医生技术的怀疑和对治疗的不理解，导致错失了原本大好的治疗时机，这样的事例在现实生活中比比皆是。就拿故事中的徐元正来说，如果他们当时没有听邻居的劝告，仍旧不相信韩医生的医术，那么徐元正的病继续拖下去还会痊愈吗？有可能等待他的将是在床上度过余生。

Han Yifeng Treats Apoplexy with Acupuncture

Han Yifeng, a county magistrate in the Qing Dynasty, was proficient in medical skills. He often diagnosed and treated diseases for people in his spare time, so his medical skills were widely spread.

Once, a local official named Xu Yuanzheng was seriously ill with symptoms of swollen face, salivated mouth, slurred speech due to blockage of the throat, heavy legs that seemed to be tied with a thousand pounds of stone and were unable to lift up and even to cross the low threshold at home. His family immediately asked Han Yifeng to treat him. After taking the pulse, Han Yifeng said to his family, "This disease must be treated by acupuncture." Han Yifeng asked the entourage to bring a candlestick and put it near the patient's head. He took out the silver needle and burned it red to prepare for the acupuncture. The official and his grandson were frightened and repeatedly refused to be needled. They said, "How can you use fire needles here? It's too dangerous to needle like this." Han Yifeng explained to the patient and his family that this treatment was safe but in vain. They still refused the treatment and Han Yifeng had to leave.

A few days later, Xu Yuanzheng's disease became worsened. One day, his neighbor came to visit him and suggested," I heard that the county magistrate Han Yifeng is skilled at acupuncture. Almost all the people in the county come to him for treatment. You can invite him to treat the disease." Hearing this, the family invited Han Yifeng again to diagnose the disease for Xu Yuanzheng. Han Yifeng did not mind their previous suspicion and diagnosed the disease carefully. He used fire needles to prick the Baihui, Shenting, Shenshu, Mingmen, Huantiao, Fengshi, Shousanli, Yongquan acupoint and other acupoints, amounting to 21 in total. At the same time, Han Yifeng arranged people to decoct medicinal herbs. The patient originally thought that the needling would be very painful before the treatment. When the needling was over, the patient was surprised pleasantly and said that it was not only painless but also comfortable to smell the aroma of the decoction. After this treatment, Xu Yuanzheng's symptoms disappeared along with the previous minor ailments.

This short story tells us that in the process of communication between people, we should learn to build a bridge of "trust". The treatment of disease is also a process of communication between doctors and patients. Some patients miss the good opportunity for disease treatment due to doubt about the doctor's skills and ignorance of the treatment, which can often be seen in real life. Take Xu Yuanzheng in the above story as an example, if he hadn't listened to the advice of his neighbor, he would not have trusted Han Yifeng's medical skills. Then how could Xu Yuanzheng's disease be cured? It is possible that he had to spend the rest of his life in bed.

有关针灸的成语

的成语

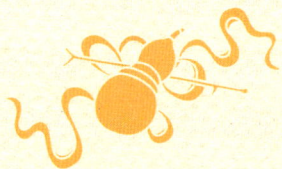

三年之艾

　　"三年之艾"出自《孟子·离娄上》："今之欲王者，犹七年之病求三年之艾也。"这本是孟子借艾与疾病的关系谈治国之道的，意思是现在想称王于天下，就像已经病了七年之久，才想起要用三年陈艾来治疗疾病。比喻凡事要平时做好准备，事到临头再想办法就来不及了。

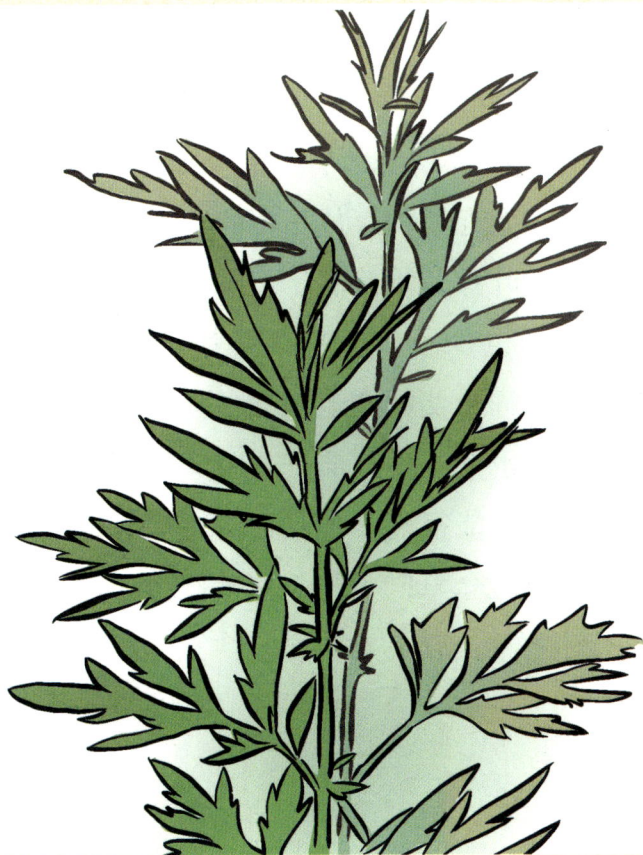

孟子向来主张仁政，认为得民心者得天下。他总结夏朝和商朝两个王朝之所以走向灭亡，是因为两朝国王夏桀和商纣都施行暴政，对待百姓十分残酷，失去了百姓的信任和拥护，老百姓一起反对他们时，他们一定会垮台的。而统一天下是有途径的，就是顺从百姓的心，多看看百姓需要什么，以人民福祉为导向，多施行仁政，他们所厌恶的就不能强加施行，那么其他国家百姓也会归附，如此一统天下的日子指日可待。

艾灸是中医非常古老的调理治疗方法，民间有谚语道："家有三年艾，郎中不用来。"艾草为菊科植物，属纯阳之品，能够激发人体阳气，祛除寒邪，增强机体免疫力和抵抗力，预防瘟疫等传染病。艾叶离人们并不遥远，端午挂艾、做艾糍、艾叶煮水泡脚和泡澡都是人们所熟知的。同时，艾叶作为一味中药，既能够内服也可以外用。一般入汤剂多用新鲜艾叶，灸疗多用陈放多年的艾叶。《本草纲目》记载："凡用艾叶，需用陈久者，治令细软，谓之熟艾，若生艾灸火，则伤人肌脉。"意思是说存放三年的艾叶用来做灸法疗效最好，超过或低于三年的艾叶疗效均降低。三年陈艾中挥发油较少，燃烧后火力持久温和，烟也少，关键是穿透力强，可以深入经络脏腑，有很好的疗效。而新鲜的艾叶含有较多的叶油，具有挥发性，燃烧时火力猛烈，冒的烟也浓，不仅会产生有害物质，对皮肤和经络也有损伤，且通达经络功能很弱。现代研究也发现，三年陈艾黄酮含量最高，过了三年峰值会急剧下降，影响疗效。所以，人们常备三年陈艾，以备不时之需。后来人们便用"三年之艾"这个成语比喻凡事必须先做准备。

The Moxa of Three Years

The idiom of "the moxa of three years" comes from *Mencius • Liloushang*: "Those who want to be the ruler of a nation are just like the patients who have been ill for seven years seeking help from the moxa of three years." Mencius applied the relationship between moxa and disease to the discussion about the way to govern a nation. The meaning is that those who want to rule a nation feel like treating a seven-year-long disease with moxa of three years. This comparison aims to remind people to make full preparations beforehand and do not wait until it is too late.

Mencius has always advocated "Benevolent Government", and held that those who win the hearts of the people win the world. He analyzed the reason for the collapse of the Xia and Shang Dynasties and concluded that the two Kings, Jie and Zhou, practiced tyranny and treated the people cruelly, thus losing the trust and support of the people. They were sure to be overthrown when the people opposed them together. The proper way to unify the country is to listen and conform to the wills of the people. Try to satisfy needs of the people, improve well-being of the people, carry out benevolent administration, and avoid imposing anything that the people dislike, and then the people of other countries will come over and pay allegiance, and the day of unifying the country can be expected soon.

Moxa-wool moxibustion is a health cultivation and treatment method of traditional Chinese medicine with a long history. A folk proverb says, "It is unnecessary to invite a doctor home if you have moxa of three years." Wormwood, as a plant in the Compositae family pertaining to pure Yang, can stimulate Yang Qi of the human body, dispel cold pathogen, enhance the organic immunity and resistance, and prevent the epidemic infectious disease and other infectious diseases. Argy wormwood leaves are not far away from our lives. We are familiar with the custom of hanging argy wormwood leaves above doorways on the Dragon Boat Festival, making glutinous rice dumplings, soaking feet and bathing with argy wormwood leaves. At the same time, as a medicinal herb, argy wormwood leaves can be taken internally and applied externally. Generally speaking, fresh argy wormwood leaves are used in decoction, and the old ones are used as moxa in moxibustion. It is recorded in *Compendium of Materia Medica records*: "Whenever argy wormwood leaves are used, the old ones are preferred. Make them fine and soft before using and they are called processed moxa. The fresh ones, if used in moxibustion, may damage the muscle and blood vessel." This indicates that the argy wormwood leaves of three years have the best efficacy for moxibustion, and those stored over or under three years are decreased in efficacy. For the argy wormwood leaves of three years, they contain less volatile oil, produce durable and mild heat, less smoke and great penetrating power when burning. Thus, they can reach deep into the meridians and zang-fu organs, and achieve fairly good effect. For the fresh argy wormwood leaves, they contain much more volatile oil, produce heavy heat, dense smoke, harmful substance and less penetrating power when burning. They may even bring about damage to the skin and meridians. Modern research also finds that the moxa of three years contains the highest content of flavone, which decreases sharply after three years, with lower curative effect accordingly. Therefore, people always prepare and store some moxa of three years against unexpected needs. Later, this idiom is used to mean that everything must be prepared fully beforehand.

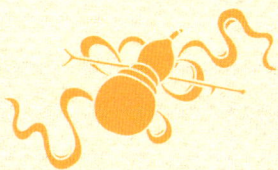

针砭时弊

　　"针砭时弊"出自南朝宋范晔所著《后汉书》："针砭时弊，月旦社会。"说的是东汉时期有位名士叫许劭，创立了"月旦评"，定期在每月初一（称为月旦）评论当时社会上的热点人物和时事，即"时弊"。这是当时的知识分子评论乡党人物，抨击社会不正之风，进而谋求社会变革进步的一种方式。在当时，如果某人想要获得辟举，入朝为官，就必须得到人们的好评。"针砭"指用针刺和砭石治病的方法，引申为指出、发现和治理错误。现在多用来形容像医生治病一样，指出时代和社会问题，劝人改正，求得向善。

　　人们谈到中医治病常常想到中药，其实还有砭、针、灸、按跷和导引等其他方法。砭石作为最原始的医疗工具，出现于距今4000~8000年前的新石器时代。《说文解字》载："砭，以石刺病也。"其最早用于刺激穴位、按摩经络、切割脓肿、刺泻瘀血，而后逐渐发展为针刺放血疗法。在古代，东南沿海地区的气候潮湿，瘴气四

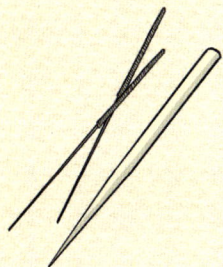

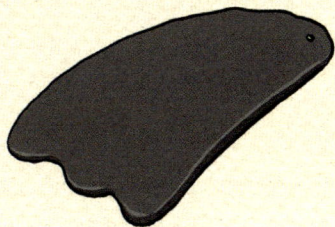

溢，人们易罹患疮疡痈疖等皮肤疾病。先民们在与这些疾病斗争的过程中发现，患处如果被尖锐的石块碰破，病情就会好转，于是人们便有意识地将石头打磨成尖锐的石器用以治疗疾病。

随着人类文明的演变，古人掌握了打磨加工技术，他们把棍棒、竹子、蚌壳、骨头、石器磨制为细长器具，虽然粗糙，但已经具有雏形。由于疾病内外深浅不一，经过不断改进，古人设计了"九针"，分别是镵针、圆针、锃针、锋针、铍针、圆利针、毫针、长针和大针，制造精巧。由于它们有九种不同的形状，在治疗上不但保留了砭石切肿排脓的功能，还极大地扩展了适用范围，随之各种刺法也逐渐形成和完善。

我们的祖先在与大自然斗争的同时，积累了大量宝贵的中医药经验与文化财富，他们的聪明才智使得我们今天的中医药事业能继续更好地为人类健康服务，我们应该好好学习传承，并将之发扬光大。

Needle Social Ills

This idiom comes from *History of the Later Han Dynasty* written by Fan Ye of the Song Dynasty during the Southern Dynasties: "Needle social ills and comment on the social issues on the day of Yuedan (Yuedan refers to the first day of every month)." This record is about a famous scholar named Xu Shao in the Eastern Han Dynasty, who started "Yuedan Review", namely giving comment on hot spots and figures of society and pointing out the problems on the first day of every month (Yuedan), which is called "social ill". It is regarded as a way for intellectuals at that time to assail social injustices by commenting on rural party figures with the purpose to seek for social reform and progress. At that time, those who wanted to be recommended and promoted to a position in the court need to be highly praised. Probing with stone needle originally refers to an ancient acupuncture method with stone needle to treat disease. By extension, it refers to pointing out, finding and correcting errors. Now the idiom is often used to describe the pointing out of problems of the times and society and the persuading of people to correct and become better in virtue.

When we talk about TCM treatment, we often think of medicinal herbs. In fact, there are many other methods such as stone needle, acupuncture, moxibustion, pressing and stamping manipulation and daoyin. The stone needle ("Bianshi" in Chinese), as the most primitive medical tools, appeared in the Neolithic Age from 4000 to 8000 years ago. The book *Library Theory and Practice* states, "Bian means to needle the diseased part with stone. It was first used to stimulate acupoints, massage meridians, cut abscesses, and expel blood stasis, and then gradually developed into blood-letting therapy with needling. In ancient times, the climate of the southeast coast was humid and miasma was prevalent. People were susceptible to skin diseases such as furuncles and carbuncle. In the process of fighting against these diseases, people found that if the affected area was broken by sharp stones, the condition could be improved. Accordingly, people consciously polished stones into sharp stone tools to treat diseases.

With the evolution of human civilization, ancient people mastered the grinding and processing technology. They ground sticks, bamboo, clam shells, bones and stones into delicate tools, which had already taken shape though still being rough. Due to the irregular depth of diseases, these tools were developed into well-designed "nine classical needles", namely shear needle, round-point needle, spoon needle, lance needle, stiletto needle, round-sharp needle, filiform needle, long needle and big needle. With nine different shapes, the nine needles not only retained the cutting function of needle stone to remove swelling and pus, but also greatly expanded the range of applications. Subsequently, various acupuncture methods were gradually formed and perfected.

While fighting against nature, our ancestors have accumulated valuable medical experience for us to deal with diseases. Their wisdom enables Chinese medicine to serve human health better. We should try our best to learn, inherit and carry it forward.

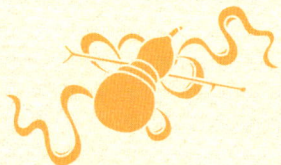

一针见血

　　"一针见血"出自南朝宋范晔《后汉书·郭玉传》："一针即瘥。"本意为一针刺下去就见到血,形容医生医术十分高明。后来比喻说话直截了当,切中要害。

　　东晋时期名臣陶侃与"一针见血"的故事有关。陶侃,字士行,浔阳人。陶侃幼年丧父,由母亲抚养成人。母亲总是以恩威并重的方式教导他,这种方式对陶侃日后成为清廉的官员有着深远的影响。传说有一次,陶侃如厕时遇见一位身穿红衣、包着头巾的人,预言

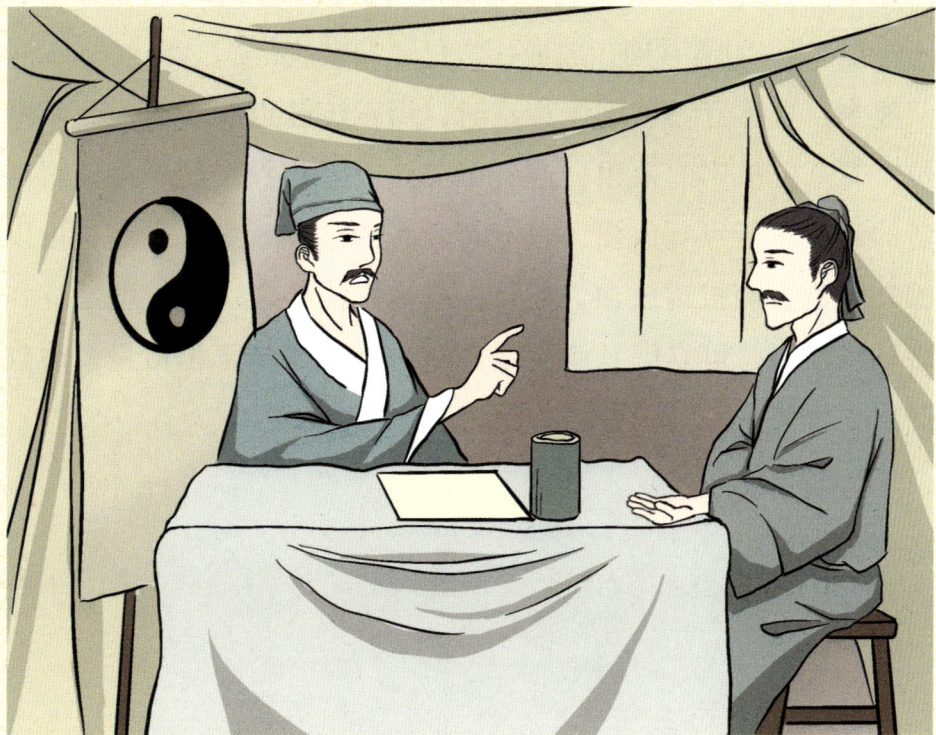

陶侃将来可以官至八州都督。又有一次，一个精通看相的人，见到陶侃左手中指有一条垂直的指纹，便说陶侃将来会做地位非常尊贵的高官，会得到"公"的爵位。听闻此言，陶侃便用针将手指刺破，喷洒到墙壁上的鲜血居然形成了一个"公"字。后来陶侃果真当了八州的都督。"一针见血"这个成语就从这里演变而出，但已和此典故无关，转用字面意思，意为一针下去，血即流出，用来形容言语简洁透彻，深中肯綮。

我们的祖国医学博大精深，其中针刺疗法就讲究一针见血，稳、准、效！在针灸时，医生要气匀神定，注意力集中，一针下去要针到病所，准确扎入穴位，达到治疗效果。在针灸中还有一种治疗方法叫放血疗法，在特定部位或者穴位上用三棱针点刺放出适量血液，通过放血祛除邪气而达到疏通经络、调和气血、平衡阴阳的治疗目的。《新唐书》记载：唐代御医用头顶放血法，治愈了唐高宗的"头眩不能视证"。明清时期，放血疗法已经非常流行。

现今，当感冒嗓子疼痛难忍时，用三棱针点刺少商、商阳两个穴位，有立竿见影的效果；遇到偏头疼或者睑腺炎的患者，可以在患者的耳尖进行点刺放血，也有奇效；如果患者出现高热，可以在大椎穴附近点刺拔罐放血。此外，放血疗法也适用于一些急症，当患者脑溢血时，可立即针刺手指十宣穴，减少脑部出血量，达到醒脑开窍的效果。总之，针刺放血的应用十分广泛。

Hit the Nail on the Head

The idiom "hit the nail on the head" comes from the phrase "to cure disease with one needle" from the book named *History of the Later Han Dynasty • Biography of Guo Yu* written by Fan Ye in the Song Dynasty during the period of Southern Dynasties. Originally, it is used to indicate the superb skill of a doctor who can draw blood with one prick. Later, it is used to describe a way of speaking which can go straight to the heart of the matter.

This idiom is related to a famous official named Tao Kan in the Eastern Jin Dynasty, who was styled Shi Xing and came from Xunyang. Tao Kan's father died when he was young, and he was brought up by his mother, who guided him with both kindness and severity. This had a profound influence on Tao Kan for his being free from corruption in his career. Legend has it that Tao Kan saw a man dressed in red with a turban when he was in the washroom. The man said that he would become governor of eight states in the future. Another time, a fortune-teller also said that he had a vertical fingerprint on the middle finger of his left hand, which was a sign to show his status would be as noble and lofty as a duke (namely "Gong" in Chinese) in the future. Tao Kan did not believe it, so he pricked his finger with a needle and the blood sprayed on the wall, forming the Chinese character "Gong" (meaning Duke). Later, Tao Kan did become a governor of the eight states. This is the story about the idiom "hit the nail on the head". Presently, it is used either to indicate its literal meaning of bleeding with needling, or to indicate the conciseness and clarity of language.

Chinese medicine is extensive and profound, among which

acupuncture therapy is particularly about hitting the nail on the head, i.e., to treat with stable, accurate and effective needling methods. In acupuncture and moxibustion, the doctor should be concentrated and calm, inserting the needle accurately to the diseased part and acupoint to achieve the expected therapeutic effect. There is also a treatment method called blood letting therapy, which aims to let out blood and expel pathogens by needling specific parts or acupoints with three-edged needles with the purpose to dredge meridians, harmonize qi and blood, balance Yin and Yang. According to the *New Book of Tang's History*, the imperial doctor of Tang Dynasty cured "the blindness caused by dizziness" of Emperor Gaozong of Tang by letting blood from the top of his head. Blood letting therapy was very popular in the Ming and Qing Dynasties.

Nowadays, sore throat due to cold can be treated by pricking Shaoshang and Shangyang acupoint with three-edged needle effectively. Migraine and hordeolum can be treated by pricking the ear tip to let blood effectively. High fever can be treated by pricking and cupping the Dazhui point to let blood. In addition, blood letting therapy is widely used for some acute syndrome like cerebral hemorrhage. Shixuan acupoint on the finger can be needled to relieve brain bleeding and induce resuscitation in this case.

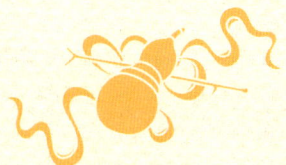

十指连心

　　"十指连心"出自明代许仲琳的小说《封神演义》第七回："十指连心，可怜昏死在地。"意思是十个手指头都连着心脏，伤着哪一个都疼，表示身体的每个小部分都与心脏有着不可分割的关系。后来比喻一个人和某人或某事具有极密切的关系。

　　春秋战国时期，儒家思想的代表人物曾子是一个有名的大孝子。

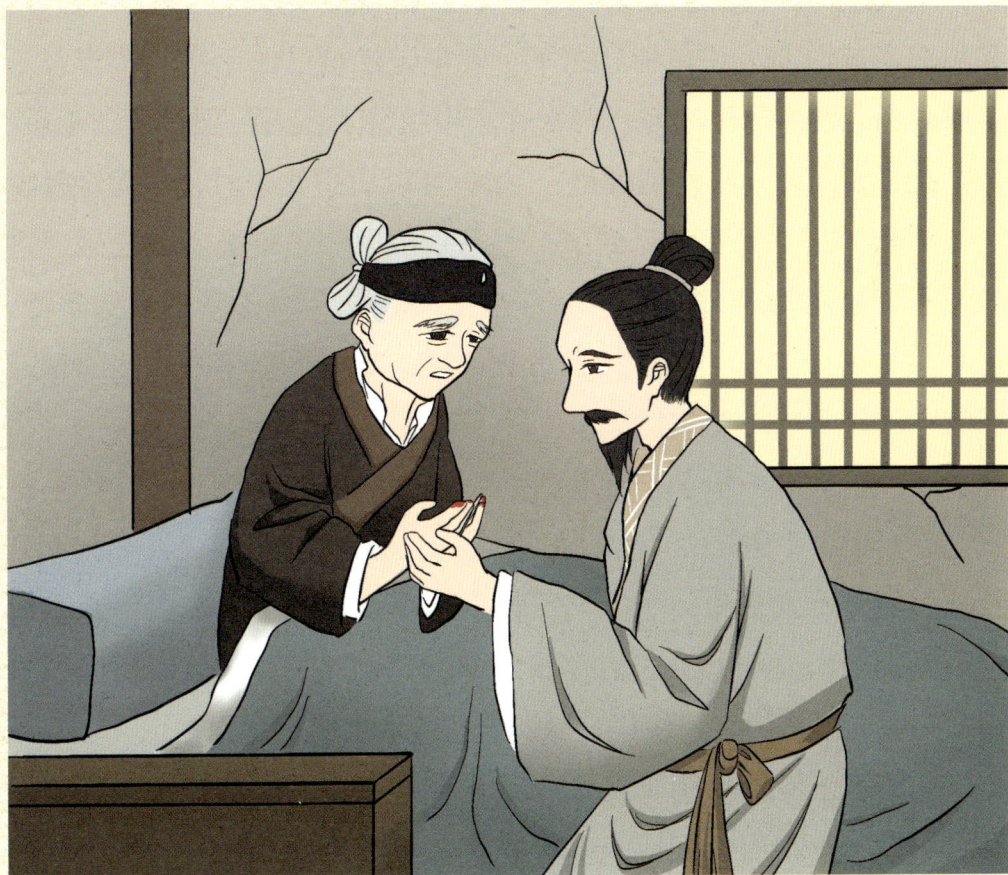

曾子小时候家境异常贫困，他父亲种地，母亲给别人做针线活，他自己只能靠上山砍柴的微薄收入贴补家用，一家三口过着清贫的生活。有一年冬天，屋外狂风呼啸凛冽，曾子把家里仅有的粮食做了一碗粥，端给抱病在床的母亲吃了，自己只能把刷锅水囫囵喝了下去。可是刷锅水根本填不饱肚子，曾子饿得肚子咕咕叫，为了不让母亲因听到自己饥肠辘辘的声音而担忧伤心，他便以上山砍柴为由躲了出去。母亲看外面天冷风大，怕他上山砍柴有危险，不让他去。曾子安慰母亲一番，搓搓带着冻疮的手，拿起砍柴刀便出门了。曾子砍到一半突然觉得心口一阵疼痛，他担心家中生病的母亲是不是出了什么事情，便赶紧收了柴刀，背起砍好的柴往山下跑。到家一看，原来是一位远房亲戚来到了曾子家中，曾母有病在身不便起身，又怕在亲戚面前失礼，情急之下，曾母咬烂自己的手指，希望曾子能感受到，然后尽快回家。曾子在家中款待了客人，把客人送走后，他跪在母亲床前，心疼地说道："娘，您以后想儿子时，只需轻轻咬一下手指，儿子就能感受到了，千万别用力咬了，更不能咬破，这样儿子会心疼的。"周围人知道了曾子的做法，纷纷赞扬他的孝行。这个小故事，体现了曾子身上难能可贵的品格——孝顺。他的孝道影响中国数千年，流传至今。

中医认为每一根手指都通过经络与相应脏腑连接，而这些脏腑又与心相通。中医认为心是"君主之官"，为五脏六腑之大主。人体有一组经外奇穴，名为十宣穴，位于十个手指的尖端，指甲游离缘附近，点刺出血可以用于治疗小儿惊厥、煤气中毒、癫病和中风急救，平时两手指尖相互碰撞，可调神益脑，增强记忆力。

大拇指上有手太阴肺经走行，与肺脏相通，揉按或放血可治疗感冒咳嗽；食指有手阳明大肠经走行，按摩可改善便秘、腹胀；中指有手厥阴心包经走行，与心包及周围组织相对应；无名指有手少阳三焦经走行，胸腹腔内所有器官不适均可揉按；小指有手少阴心经和手太阳小肠经走行，对应心和小肠，"心主神明"，刺激小手指内侧能够宁心安神，有助睡眠。另外，手指出现的一些症状也能够反映出心脏的病变。比如，手指端呈杵状，是长期心肺疾病导致身体慢性缺氧的表现；指甲苍白、外翻呈反杓状，是长期气血亏虚未得到纠正的表现；一些心肌梗死患者发病时，会表现出手指麻木和疼痛。

The Fingers are Linked to the Heart

The idiom "the fingers are linked to the heart" comes from the seventh chapter of the novel *The Investiture of the Gods* written by Xu Zhonglin in the Ming Dynasty. It says, "Since the ten fingers are linked to the heart, he fell to the ground in a dead faint." The phrase means that all the ten fingers are connected to the heart, and it hurts if any one of them is injured. It indicates that every small part of the body has an inseparable relationship with the heart. Later, this idiom is used to show the close relationship between people or things.

In the Spring and Autumn Period and the Warring States Period, Zeng Zi, a representative figure of Confucianism, was a famous filial son. When he was young, his family was very poor and made a living by doing some farm work, sewing work and cutting firewood. On a cold and windy winter day, Zeng Zi made a bowl of porridge with the only grain for his sick mother in bed, and he himself could only gulp down the pot-washing water, which was of course unable to relieve his hunger. To let his mother free from worrying about his hunger, he planned to go up the mountain to cut firewood. His mother, thinking of the cold weather and potential danger, was unwilling to let him go. Zeng Zi comforted her and left home with a machete in his frostbitten hand. In the process of cutting firewood, he felt painful in the heart suddenly and was worried that something must have happened to his mother. So he quickly ran back home with the firewood collected, and found that there was a distant relative coming to visit them. His mother, being unable to get up due to the disease, was afraid of being impolite in front of the relative, so she bitted through her finger with the hope of letting Zeng Zi feel it. Zeng Zi treated the guest well and sent him away. He knelt by his mother's bed and said, "Mom, if you miss me from now on, you just bite your finger gently and then I can feel it. Don't bite so hard, otherwise my heart would be broken." When the people around heard the story, they praised him highly for his filial piety. The valuable filial piety of Zeng Zi has exerted great influence in China for thousands of years and has been passed down till now.

Traditional Chinese medicine (TCM) believes that each finger is connected to the corresponding zang-fu organs through the meridians, which are further connected to the heart. The heart is called "the monarch organ" in TCM, and governs the zang-fu organs. There is a type of acupoints located at the end of the ten fingers and near the nails, which are called Shixuan acupoint. The general puncture bleeding method can be used to treat infantile convulsion, carbon monoxide poisoning, hysteria and stroke. In daily life, people can knock the fingertips with each other to enhance memory by regulating the spirit and benefiting the brain.

The Taiyin Lung Meridian of Hand circulates along the thumb and connects with the lung. Kneading or bloodletting it can treat cough caused by cold. The Yangming Large Intestine Meridian of Hand circulates along the index finger, and massage of it can treat constipation and abdominal distension. The Jueyin Pericardium Meridian of Hand circulates along the middle finger and corresponds to the pericardium and surrounding tissues. The Shaoyang Sanjiao Meridian of Hand circulates along the ring finger and kneading it can relieve the disorders of all the organs in the chest and abdomen. The Shaoyin Heart Meridian of Hand and the Taiyang Small Intestine Meridian of Hand circulate along the little finger, which corresponds to the heart and the small intestine. Since the heart is believed to govern the spirit and mental activities in TCM, kneading the little finger can calm the mind and benefit sleep. In addition, some symptoms of fingers can also reflect the heart disease. For example, clubbing finger indicates chronic oxygen deficiency due to diseases of the heart or lung. Pale and everted nail indicates long-term deficiency of qi and blood. Numbness and pain of the fingers may indicate the occurrence of myocardial infarction.

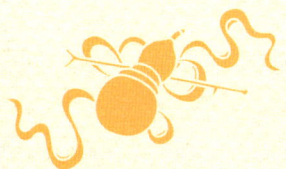

灼艾分痛

　　"灼艾分痛"出自《宋史·太祖本纪》，讲的是宋太祖赵匡胤与弟弟宋太宗赵光义之间兄弟友爱的故事。

　　宋太祖赵匡胤生于 927 年，卒于 976 年，公元 960 年在"陈桥兵变"后登基为帝，定国号为"宋"，史称宋朝或北宋。赵匡胤智慧超人、善良温暖、宽容仁慈，是一位深受朝中大臣和黎民百姓拥护爱戴的皇帝。赵匡胤有一个弟弟，名叫赵光义，即后来的宋太宗。

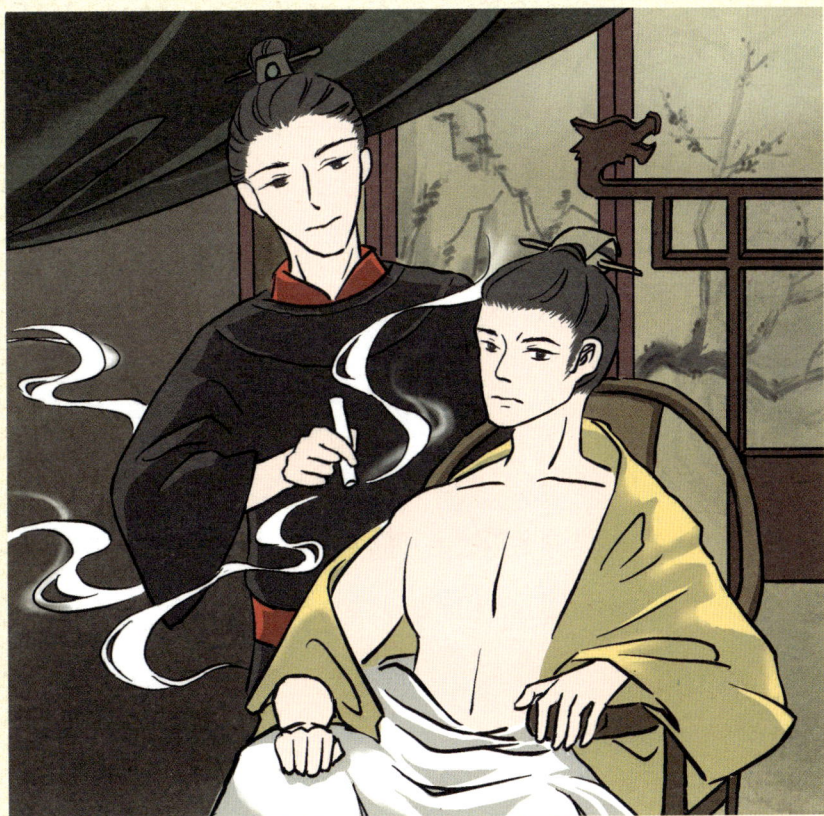

兄弟俩同是昭宪太后杜氏所生。赵匡胤对赵光义疼爱有加，甚至将皇位传给他。这种兄弟情深、超然大度的品格一直被传为佳话。

有一天，弟弟赵光义得了非常严重的疾病，多日卧床不起，常常腹中疼痛难忍、茶饭不思、手足厥冷、浑身无力，太医院的大夫为他诊病后，认为用艾灸治疗效果最好。宋太祖听说弟弟重病缠身，十分关心，忙完政务后便立即赶到弟弟家中探望。刚一进门，就听见弟弟哀声连连，拒绝艾灸。宋太祖看在眼里，疼在心上，他接过大夫手上的艾绒，亲自为弟弟施灸，然而宋太宗依然痛苦难耐，嚎啕大哭。宋太祖为了安慰弟弟，让他配合治疗，便将艾绒对准自己的皮肤烧灼起来，以亲身感受弟弟的痛楚。弟弟看到哥哥为自己所做的一切，十分感动，便咬紧牙关，接受了艾灸的治疗，不久就病愈了。后来人们以"灼艾分痛"记载这个故事，多用来形容兄弟间的友爱之情。

艾灸的出现最早可追溯到远古时期，是中国最古老的医术之一。此疗法不仅在民间广为流传，也深得王公贵族的喜爱。有人或许会疑惑，为什么太宗艾灸那么痛苦，与现代平时看到的艾灸不太一样呢？这是因为在古代瘢痕灸较为盛行。瘢痕灸也称化脓灸，操作时先在施术部位涂少量大蒜汁，再放上点燃的艾炷，等待艾炷燃尽后换个艾炷再灸。这种施灸方法灼伤较重，可使局部皮肤溃破、化脓，留下永久瘢痕，多用来治疗一些疑难病症。宋太宗病情严重，从其施灸时的反应来看，推测是采用了瘢痕灸。艾灸疗法种类繁多，针对不同疾病应遵医嘱选用适宜疗法，以达到祛病强身、延年益寿的功效。

Burning Moxa to Share Pain

This idiom, recorded in the *History of Song Dynasty • Biography of Taizu*, is about the story between Zhao Kuangyin, Taizu of the Song Dynasty, and his younger brother Zhao Guangyi, Taizong of the Song Dynasty.

Zhao Kuangyin was born in 927 and died in 976. He became emperor in 960 after the Chenqiao Mutiny. The title of his kingdom was Song, which is known as the Song or Northern Song Dynasty in history. Zhao Kuangyin was a wise, kind, warm, lenient and benevolent king, who was supported and loved by the ministers and people greatly. He had a younger brother named Zhao Guangyi, who later became Emperor Taizong of Song. They were children of Empress Dowager Zhao Xian surnamed Du. Zhao Kuangyin loved his brother dearly and even gave him the throne. His affection for his brother and magnanimous character have long been well-known.

One day, Zhao Guangyi got a very serious disease and was bedridden for several days with symptoms of abdominal pain, poor appetite, reversal cold of hands and feet, weakness and fatigue. The doctor from Imperial Hospital diagnosed that moxa-wool moxibustion could be used to treat his disease. When Zhao Kuangyin heard his brother was seriously ill, he rushed to visit his brother at home immediately after he finished his government affairs. He saw that his brother was crying non-stop and refusing moxibustion as he entered the room. Caring his brother so much, he took over moxa and carried out moxibustion for his brother in person. However, his brother was still painful and cried bitterly. In order to encourage his brother to cooperate with the treatment, Zhao Kuangyin burned the moxa wool on his own skin to feel his brother's pain. The younger brother was very touched, so he clenched his teeth to continue the moxa-wool moxibustion and recovered soon. Later, people documented this story with the idiom "burning moxa to share pain" to describe the brotherly love.

As one of the oldest medical skills in China, the origin of moxa-wool moxibustion can be traced back to ancient times. It was very popular among the common people and the noble and royal as well. Some people may wonder why the moxa-wool moxibustion of Taizong was so painful, which is quite different with that commonly seen nowadays. This is because he might be treated with scarring moxibustion that was popular in ancient times. Scarring moxibustion is also known as suppurative moxibustion. It is performed by applying a small amount of garlic juice on the diseased body part, then puting the lit moxa cone, waiting for the moxa cone to burn out, and then changeing a new one. This moxibustion method burns the skin seriously, which often leads to dermal rupture, fester and permanent cicatrices, so it is used to treat some difficult and complicated diseases. During Taizong of the Song Dynasty's serious illness, it was suspected that scarring moxibustion was used, based on his reaction when moxibustion was applied. There are various kinds of moxa-wool moxibustion therapies, and they should be selected properly to treat different diseases directed by the doctors to dispel disease, preserve health and prolong life.